Problem Solving:

Physical Pharmacy

Problem Solving:

Physical Pharmacy

Alfred Martin, Ph.D.
Emeritus Coulter R. Sublett Professor
Drug Dynamics Institute
College of Pharmacy
University of Texas
Austin, Texas

Pilar Bustamante, Ph.D.
Titular Professor
Department of Pharmacy
and Pharmaceutical Technology
Facultad de Farmacia
University of Alcalá de Henares
Madrid, Spain

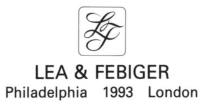

LEA & FEBIGER
Philadelphia   1993   London

Lea & Febiger
Box 3024
200 Chester Field Parkway
Malvern, Pennsylvania 19355-9725
U.S.A.
(610) 251-2230

PRINTED IN THE UNITED STATES OF AMERICA

Print Number: 5 4 3 2

Preface

Problem Solving: Physical Pharmacy is a bridge between the theoretical principles in *Physical Pharmacy, 4th ed.,* and the problems encountered by the pharmacist in practice, research and dosage formulation. The purpose of this manual is to help the readers of *Physical Pharmacy, 4th ed.,* carry out the calculations required in solving the problems in each chapter. By working the problems, students, researchers and pharmacists get a better understanding of the concepts and principles presented in each chapter. The problems also bring the student's attention to the use of proper units and dimensions. Failure to express a quantity in the proper units will lead to wrong answers.

Most of the new problems are based on papers published in pharmaceutical journals. Some problems also use data from journals in the basic sciences, for example, those from the fields of colloids and powder technology. Pharmacy is an applied science and principles from other areas are used in the design and stabilization of drugs. In some cases the data for a problem is modified or read directly from the figure in the published paper and may differ somewhat from the results given in the original article.

In this manual the worked problems follow the ordering of chapters and problems found in *Physical Pharmacy, 4th ed.* Figures and tables in the problem solving manual are given a binary notation referring to the Chapter and problem number. The figures and tables in the manual also contain a P (which stands for problem solving manual) to avoid confusion when referring to the tables or figures of *Physical Pharmacy, 4th ed.* For example, Table P12-7 is the seventh table in Chapter 12 in the manual whereas Table 12-7 refers to the seventh table of Chapter 12 in *Physical Pharmacy, 4th ed.*

In regression analysis as many digits as are available in the calculator or computer are carried in the computation. Rounding off of digits is postponed until the final step in most cases. The student's results may differ slightly from those found in the text depending on the stage and the degree of roundoff. The student may also obtain slightly different answers from those in the book by using, for example, 273°K versus 273.15°K for 0°C, or 18 gram/mole versus 18.015 gram/mole for the molecular weight of water.

We wish to thank Dr. Stephan F. Baron, of Leeds and Northrup, for checking the authors' calculations of the problems. Alfred Martin is grateful to Dean J. T. Doluisio and his colleagues for their advice and support and to Coulter R. Sublett for the emeritus professorship generously provided in his name. Pilar Bustamante kindly thanks Dr. Selles and her colleagues in the Department of Pharmacy and Pharmaceutical Technology (Alcalá de Henares, Madrid) for their support and encouragement. We also wish to thank Thomas Colaiezzi, George H. Mundorff and John F. Spahr, Jr. of Lea & Febiger for supporting the idea of the manual, *Problem Solving: Physical Pharmacy* and for putting it into finished form.

Alfred Martin, Austin, Texas
Pilar Bustamante, Madrid, Spain

Contents

CHAPTER 1
Introduction

PROBLEM 1.1. The SI units corresponding to g/cm^3 is kg/m^3

$$\rho = 2.23\frac{g}{cm^3} \times \frac{1kg}{10^3 g} \times \frac{(10^2)^3 cm^3}{1m^3} = 2.23 \times 10^3 \frac{kg}{m^3}$$

PROBLEM 1.2. $1\ nm = 10^{-9}\ m$; $1\ cm = 10^{-2}\ m$

$$2.736\ nm \times \frac{10^{-9}\ m}{1\ nm} \times \frac{1\ cm}{10^{-2}\ m} = 2.736 \times 10^{-7}\ cm$$

PROBLEM 1.3. $1\ nm = 10^{-9}\ m$; $1\ \text{Å} = 10^{-8}\ cm = 10^{-10}\ m$

$$1\ \text{Å} = 10^{-10}\ m \times \frac{1\ nm}{10^{-9}\ m} = 0.1\ nm;\quad 1.99 \times 10^4\ \text{Å}^3 = (1.99 \times 10^4)(0.1)^3\ nm^3$$

$$= 19.9\ nm^3$$

PROBLEM 1.4. $1\ \text{dyne} = 1\ g\ \dfrac{cm}{sec^2}$; $\dfrac{1\ dyne}{cm} = \dfrac{1\ g}{sec^2}$

$$27.32\ \frac{g}{sec^2} \times \frac{10^{-3}\ kg}{g} = 0.02732\ kg\ sec^{-2} = 0.02723\ N\ m^{-1}$$

(Since $N = m\ kg\ sec^{-2}$; $N\ m^{-1} = kg\ sec^{-2}$)
$N\ m = J$; $N = J\ m^{-1}$
$0.02732\ N\ m^{-1} = 0.02732\ J\ m^{-1}\ m^{-1} = 0.02732\ J\ m^{-2}$

PROBLEM 1.5. $259\ cal \times \dfrac{4.1840\ J}{cal} = 1084\ J$

PROBLEM 1.6. $1\ erg = 1\ g\ cm^2\ sec^{-2}$;

$$3.8 \times 10^{11}\ g\ cm^2\ sec^{-2} \times \frac{1\ kg}{1000\ g} \times \frac{1\ m^2}{100^2\ cm^2} = 3.8 \times 10^{11} \times 10^{-7}\ \frac{kg\ m^2}{sec^2}$$

$$= 3.8 \times 10^4\ kg\ m^2\ sec^{-2}$$

PROBLEM 1.7. $8.3143\ J\ {}^\circ K^{-1}\ mole^{-1}\ \dfrac{1\ cal}{4.184\ J} = \dfrac{8.3143}{4.184}\ cal\ {}^\circ K^{-1}\ mole^{-1}$

$$= 1.9872\ cal\ {}^\circ K^{-1}\ mole^{-1}$$

PROBLEM 1.8. $1 \text{ N m}^{-2} = 1 \text{ Pa}$; $50{,}237 \text{ Pa} = 50{,}237 \text{ N m}^{-2}$;

$$50{,}237 \text{ N/m}^2 \times \frac{1 \ atm}{101{,}325N \ m^{-2}} = \frac{50{,}237}{101{,}325} \text{ atm}$$

$$\frac{50{,}237}{101{,}325} \ atm \times \frac{760 \ torrs}{1 \ atm} = 376.8 \text{ torrs}$$

PROBLEM 1.9. $1 \text{ erg} = \text{cm}^2 \text{ g sec}^{-2}$; $1 \text{ J} = \text{m}^2 \text{ kg sec}^{-2}$

$$4.379 \times 10^6 \text{ g cm}^2 \text{ sec}^{-2} \times \frac{m^2}{10^4 \ cm^2} \times \frac{kg}{10^3 \ g} = 4.379 \ \frac{10^6}{10^7} \text{ m}^2 \text{ sec}^{-2} \text{ kg} = 0.4379 \text{ J}$$

PROBLEM 1.10. Since pressure is defined as force per unit area (dyne/cm^2), and force is mass times gravity acceleration, g.

$$\text{pressure} = \frac{force}{unit \ area \ (cm^2)} = \frac{mass \times g}{cm^2} = \frac{volume \times density \times g}{cm^2}$$

The volume is obtained by multiplying the height (h) of the mineral oil (or mercury) column (cm) times the cross section of the column, i.e., cm x cm^2 = cm^3.

$$\text{Pressure} = \frac{h \times cm^2 \times \rho \times g}{cm^2} = \text{h } \rho \text{ g dyne cm}^{-2};$$

The height of a column of mineral oil at 25 °C is

$$h = \frac{Pressure}{\rho \times g} = \frac{1.01325 \times 10^6 \ dyne/cm^2}{0.860 \ g/cm^3 \times 980.665 \ cm/sec^2} = 1201 \text{ cm}$$

$$= 1201 \text{ cm} \times 0.0328 \text{ ft/cm} = 39 \text{ ft}$$

PROBLEM 1.11. The answer is given in the problem.

PROBLEM 1.12. $\log_{5.9} (1000) = \log (1000)/\log (5.9) = 3/0.7709 = 3.8916$
$\log_{5.9} (100) = \log (100)/\log (5.9) = 2/0.7709 = 2.5944$
$\log_{5.9} (10) = \log (10)/0.7709 = 1.2972$
$\log_{5.9} (1) = \log (1)/0.7709 = 0$
$\log_{5.9} (0.1) = \log (0.1)/0.7709 = -1.2972$
$\log_{5.9} (0.001) = \log (0.001)/0.7709 = -3.8916$

PROBLEM 1.13. Since $P = k\frac{1}{V}$ and y = ax + b, the constant k is obtained from the

slope of a plot of P against 1/V. (Figure P1-1). The data needed are presented in Table P1-1. It should be noted that the slope of the line is calculated from two points selected from the

Table P1-1 for Problem 1.13.

1/V (liters^{-1})	0.0112	0.0223	0.0446	0.0893	0.1786
P (atm)	0.25	0.50	1.0	2.0	4.0

line, and not from two of the experimental points from the data. While in this problem the points fall directly on the line, such is not always the case, and the "line of best fit" must be drawn.

$$\text{slope} = \frac{\Delta y}{\Delta x} = \frac{y_2 - y_1}{x_2 - x_1}$$

Choosing the points (4.0 − 0.25), (0.1786 − 0.0112), the slope, k, is

$$k = \frac{4.0 - 0.25}{0.1786 - 0.0112} = 22.4 \text{ liter atm}$$

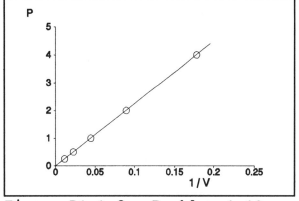

Figure P1-1 for Problem 1.13

A pressure of 1 atm is equal to the pressure exerted by a column of mercury 76 cm high and 1 cm in cross section at 0°C. It is also defined as a force per unit area (see problem 1.10).

P = h ρ g = 76 cm x 13.595 g/cm^2 x 980 cm/sec^2 = 1012555.6 dyne cm^{-2}

k = 22,400 atm cm^3 x

$$1012555.6 \frac{dyne\ cm^{-2}}{atm} = 2.2681 \times 10^{10}$$

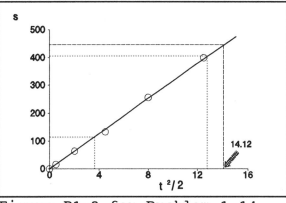

Figure P1-2 for Problem 1.14

dyne cm = 2.27 x 10^{10} erg

In joules: $\dfrac{1\ J}{10^7\ erg} = \dfrac{x}{2.27 \times 10^{10}\ erg}$; x = 2.27 x 10^3 J

In calories: $\dfrac{4.184\ J}{1\ cal} = \dfrac{2.27 \times 10^3\ J}{x\ cal}$; x = 5.43 x 10^2 cal

PROBLEM 1.14. Plotting s versus (1/2)t^2, the value of g is given by the slope of the line. The line of best fit (Figure P1-2) is drawn and the slope calculated as in problem 1.13.

$$g = \text{slope} = \frac{414 - 120}{13 - 3.8} = 32 \text{ ft/sec.}$$

Extrapolating on the graph (dashed line), the value for t^2/2 is 14.12 when s = 450 ft ;

Table P1-2 for Problem 1.14.

s	0	16	64	144	256	400
$t^2/2$	0	0.5	2.0	4.5	8.0	12.5

$t^2 = 2 \times 14.12 = 28.24 \text{ sec}^2$

$t = \sqrt{28.24} = 5.3 \text{ sec}$

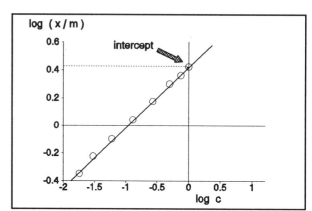

Figure P1-3 for Problem 1.15

PROBLEM 1.15. Taking logs,

$\log (x/m) = n \log c + \log k$

Plotting $\log (x/m)$ versus $\log c$, n is computed from the slope of the line and $\log k$ is the y-intercept. From Figure P1 − 3:

$n = \text{slope} = \dfrac{0.34 - (-0.31)}{-0.2 - (-1.73)} = 0.42$

The value of $\log k$ is equal to $\log (x/m)$ when $n \log c = 0$, i.e, when $c = 1$. From Figure P1 − 3:

Intercept $= \log k = 0.423$; $k = 2.65$

PROBLEM 1.16. The equation is written in logarithmic form :

$\ln k = \dfrac{E_a}{R} \dfrac{1}{T} + \ln A$

A regression of $\ln k$ against $1/T$ gives $\dfrac{E_a}{R}$ from the slope and $\ln A$ from the intercept. The data needed are shown in Table P1 − 3.

The equation is: $\ln k = -10141.07 \dfrac{1}{T} + 30.0536$; $r = -0.9986$; $r^2 = 0.9973$

Table P1 − 3 for Problem 1.16.

lnk	T (°K)	1/T x 10^3 °K^{-1}
− 2.3026	313.15	3.1934
− 1.3863	323.15	3.0945
− 0.3567	333.15	3.0017

$A = \exp(30.0536) = 1.13 \times 10^{13}\ \text{sec}^{-1};\quad \text{slope} = -10141.07 = -\dfrac{E_a}{R}$

$E_a = 1.9872 \times 10141.07 = 20{,}152\ \text{cal/mole}$

PROBLEM 1.17 (a). Using ln G vs.

ln F, N ln F = ln η' + ln G and

ln G = N ln F − ln η'

Similarly, using log G vs. log F,

log G = N log F − log η'

The data (Table P1 − 4) are plotted in Figure P1 − 4.

From the Figure (right straight line),

$\text{slope} = \dfrac{\ln G_2 - \ln G_1}{\ln F_2 - \ln F_1}$

$= \dfrac{4 - 1}{7.57 - 6.5} = 2.80$

From Figure P1 − 4 (left straight line),

$\text{slope} = \dfrac{\log G_2 - \log G_1}{\log F_2 - \log F_1} = \dfrac{2.07 - 0.5}{3.28 - 2.71} = 2.75$

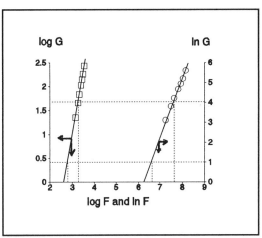

Figure P1-4 for Problem 1.17

We obtain almost the same values for N using log or ln. The small difference is due to reading from the graph.

Table P1 − 4 for Problem 1.17.

ln F (x − axis)	ln G (right y − axis)	log F (x − axis)	log G (left y − axis)
7.2605	3.1224	3.1532	1.3560
7.4978	3.8155	3.2562	1.6571
7.6411	4.2195	3.3185	1.8325
7.8232	4.6634	3.3976	2.0253
7.9413	4.9416	3.4489	2.1461
8.0353	5.1985	3.4897	2.2576
8.1605	5.6058	3.5441	2.4346

Using the data in Table P1 − 4 yields N = 2.76 in both cases (ln and log values).

(b) Figure P1 − 5 shows the direct plot of G vs F on log − log paper. To get the slope = N, we read off two values of G and two values of F and change them to log or ln. For example, we read off (157.5, 3000) and (60, 2000)

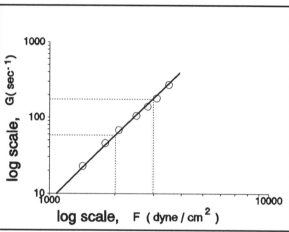

Figure P1-5 for Problem 1.17

Using log,

$$\text{slope} = \frac{\log 157.5 - \log 60}{\log 3000 - \log 2000} = 2.38$$

If we use ln, the result is the same:

$$\text{slope} = \frac{\ln 157.5 - \ln 60}{\ln 3000 - \ln 2000} = 2.38.$$

This is due to the fact that log − log paper does not distinguish between ln and log.

(c) Using log together with linear regression:

log G = 2.69 log F − 7.1018;

$r^2 = 0.9982$

N = 2.69; $\eta' = $ antilog(7.1018) = 1.26 x 10^7

Using ln together with linear regression:

ln G = 2.69 ln F − 16.3556 ; ($r^2 = 0.9982$)

N = 2.69; $\eta' = e^{16.3556} = 1.27$ x 10^7

The small difference is due to rounding off errors. Regression analysis provides better results than the graphical methods. It is hard to read off the values from the plots.

PROBLEM 1.18. The slope and intercept are calculated using regression analysis. The data are presented in Table P1 − 5.

Table P1 − 5 for Problem 1.18.

t (x)	log s (y)	ln s (y)
1	2.4138	5.5580
2	2.2833	5.2575
3	2.1532	4.9579
4	2.0228	4.6578

Using ln, ln s = 5.8579 − 0.300 t $(r^2 = 0.9999)$

s_o = exp (5.8579) = 350 km ; k = slope = 0.300 hr^{-1}

Using log, log s = 2.5441 − 0.1303 t $(r^2 = 0.9999)$

s_o = antilog (2.5441) = $10^{2.5441}$ = 350 km

k = slope x 2.303 = 0.1303 x 2.303 = 0.300 hr^{-1}

In order to get s_o we must take the antilog of the intercept in both cases. However, we obtain the k value directly from the slope using ln whereas we must multiply the slope by 2.303 when using log_{10}. There is no reason to change the data from ln to log when plotting because the log paper does not distinguish between log and ln. They are related through a proportionality constant, i. e., ln = (2.303) x (log).

PROBLEM 1.19. The data needed for the calculations are shown in Table P1 − 6. The average weight is:

$$\text{Av. wt., } \overline{x} = \frac{\sum x}{N} = \frac{17.82}{6} = 2.97 \text{ grain}$$

The average deviation is:

$$\text{Av. dev.} = \frac{\sum (x - \overline{x})}{N} = \frac{0.62}{6} = 0.103 \text{ grain}$$

The standard error for a small sample is:

$$s = \sqrt{\frac{\sum (x - \overline{x})^2}{N - 1}} = \sqrt{\frac{0.0850}{6 - 1}} = 0.13 \text{ grain}$$

Table P1 − 6 for Problem 1.19.

x	$x - \overline{x}$	$(x - \overline{x})^2$
2.85	− 0.12	0.0144
2.80	− 0.17	0.0289
3.02	0.05	0.0025
3.05	0.08	0.0064
2.95	− 0.02	0.0004
3.15	0.18	0.0324

PROBLEM 1.20. (a) Using Table 1 – 7 (Chapter 1) and an HP 41C hand calculator, $r^2 = 0.9998$; $r = 0.9999$

The equation is $y = 1.501 - (4.00 \cdot 10^{-4})x$

slope $= -4.00 \cdot 10^{-4}$; intercept $= 1.501$

(b) Using Table 1 – 8 (Chapter 1) and the least squares method, the equation of the line is log $y = 0.843 - 0.279 x$; $r^2 = 0.9986$

PROBLEM 1.21. (a) $r^2 = 0.9843$; slope $= 29.46$; intercept $= -2272$. (see Figure P1 – 6, line (a)

(b) Removing nitrobenzene from the set of data, $r^2 = 0.9599$; slope $= 26.14$; intercept $= -1255$;

(c) (1) $r^2 = 0.9914$; slope $= 24.65$; intercept $= -921.5$

(c) (2) $r^2 = 0.9810$; slope $= 24.57$; intercept $= -839$, see Figure P1 – 6, line (c)(2)

(c) (3) $r^2 = 0.9639$; slope $= 27.0$; intercept $= -1517$

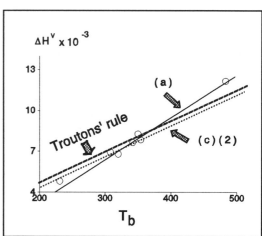

Figure P1–6 for Problem 1.21

(d) The value for the slope varies and is closer to 23 when nitrobenzene is removed. The variation of the slope shows that the least squares method is not resistant to, but rather is influenced by, extreme values (outliers). More compounds would be helpful.

PROBLEM 1.22.

(See Figure P1 – 7).

The regression equation is:

RA $= 2.472 + 0.5268$ log K;

$r^2 = 0.8262$; $r = 0.9089$

Table P1 – 7 lists the calculated activities and the % difference

= [(observed – calculated)/observed] x 100

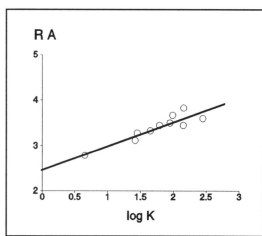

Figure P1–7 for Problem 1.22

Table P1 – 7 for Problem 1.22.

log K	Relative Activity, RA	
	Calculated	% Difference
0.6503	2.81	− 0.72
1.4200	3.22	− 3.2
2.1501	3.60	− 4.3
1.6503	3.34	− 0.3
1.4502	3.24	1.2
1.9899	3.52	4.1
2.4499	2.76	− 4.4
1.9499	3.50	0
1.7903	3.41	3.6
2.1562	3.61	5.7

PROBLEM 1.23. The regression equation is:

log (1/C) = 2.1703 + 1.0580 (log K) − 0.2226 (log K)^2; r^2 = 0.9964

A plot of log 1/C against log K shows a parabolic relationship (Figure P1 – 8). Table P1 – 8 lists the calculated 1/C values and the residuals (1/C observed − 1/C calculated).

PROBLEM 1.24. (a) The equation is:

log S = 1.3793 − 2.5201 (V/100) − 0.1216 π + 1.8148 ß; r^2 = 0.9811

(b) The predicted S values and the percent error are shown in Table P1 – 9.

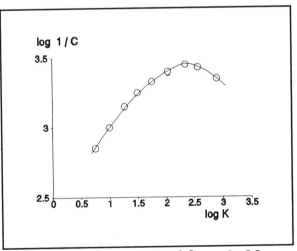

Figure P1-8 for Problem 1.23

Table P1 − 8 for Problem 1.23.

log(1/C)	2.84	3.01	3.15	3.36	3.34	3.40	3.43	3.42	3.37
Residual	0.011	−0.006	−0.005	−0.007	−0.010	−0.001	0.023	0.011	−0.017

Table P1 − 9 for Problem 1.24.

log S (calc)	1.073	0.675	0.328	0.262	−0.171	0.314	−0.087	−0.437	−0.955	−0.514
% error	5.7	2.1	0.005	−118.6	−44.77	12.7	44.3	40.8	2.6	3

PROBLEM 1.25. Figure P1 − 9 shows a plot of the data.

Quadratic equation:

$$\rho = 1.000019094 + (2.758 \times 10^{-5})\, t - (5.912 \times 10^{-6})\, t^2 \; ; \; r^2 = 0.9956$$

At 15.56 °C: $\rho = 0.99901692$ g/cm^3

At 25°C $\rho = 0.9970137$ (CRC p. F − 5 gives 0.9970479)

At 37°C $\rho = 0.9929462$ (CRC p. F − 5 gives 0.9933316)

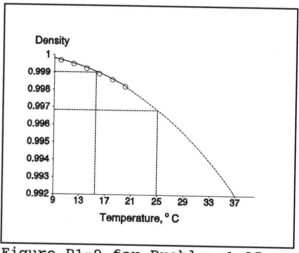

Figure P1-9 for Problem 1.25

Cubic equation:

$$\rho = 0.999870506 + (5.9 \times 10^{-5})t - (8.09 \times 10^{-6})\, t^2 + (4.8 \times 10^{-8})\, t^3$$
$$r^2 = 0.9987$$

At 25°C, $\rho = 0.9970524$ (CRC p. F − 5 gives 0.9970479)

At 37°C, $\rho = 0.9934406$ (CRC p. F − 5 gives 0.9933316)

Reading off from Figure P1 − 9, at 15.56°C, $\rho = 0.9991$. At 25°C, $\rho = 0.9968$ At 37°C, $\rho = 0.9920$

Comparison of these values with CRC values above shows that it is not safe to extrapolate graphically the results. Extrapolation using the regression equation provides much better values.

PROBLEM 1.26. Using regression analysis:

log (x/m) = 0.432 log c + 0.4240

$r^2 = 0.9989; r = 0.9995$

b = n = slope = 0.432

CHAPTER 2
States of Matter

PROBLEM 2.1. $\dfrac{P_1 V_1}{T_1} = \dfrac{P_2 V_2}{T_2}$

$$V_2 = \frac{1\ atm \times 2.5\ \ell \times 228.15\ ^\circ K}{297.15\ ^\circ K \times 8.77 \times 10^{-3}\ atm} = 219\ \text{liters}$$

PROBLEM 2.2. The volume at the bottom of the tank is:

$$V_1 = \frac{4}{3}\pi r^3 = \frac{4}{3} \times 3.1416\,(0.1)^3\ cm^3 = 4.19 \times 10^{-3}\ cm^3$$

At the surface the pressure, P_2 is $\dfrac{750}{760} = 0.99$ atm; $\quad \dfrac{P_1 V_1}{T_1} = \dfrac{P_2 V_2}{T_2}$

$$V_2 = \frac{1.3\ atm \times 4.19 \times 10^{-3}\ cm^3 \times 300.15\ ^\circ K}{0.99\ atm \times 287.15\ ^\circ K} = 5.75 \times 10^{-3}\ cm^3$$

$$5.75\ cm^3 \times 10^{-3} = \frac{4}{3} \times 3.1416 \times r^3; \quad r^3 = 1.37 \times 10^{-3}\ cm^3$$

$$r = \sqrt[3]{1.37 \times 10^{-3}} = 0.11\ \text{mm}$$

The radius is increased from 0.1 cm to 0.11 cm.

PROBLEM 2.3. $V = \dfrac{nRT}{P} =$

$$\frac{0.08205\ \ell\ atm\ mole^{-1}\ deg^{-1} \times 273.15\ deg^{-1}}{400\ atm} = 0.056\ \text{liter} = 56\ \text{ml}$$

PROBLEM 2.4. (a) $PV = nRT = \dfrac{g}{M}\ RT;\ M = \dfrac{g\,R\,T}{PV}$

$$M = \frac{0.5\ g \times 0.08205\ \ell\ atm/^\circ K\ mole \times 393.15\ ^\circ K}{1\ atm \times 0.1\ \ell} = 161\ \text{g/mole}$$

PROBLEM 2.5. (a) The molecular weight is: $M = \dfrac{gRT}{PV}$

$$M = \frac{6.07\ g \times 0.08205\ \ell\ atm/^\circ K\ mole \times 301.15\ ^\circ K}{1.17\ atm \times 2.0\ \ell} = 64.1\ \text{g/mole}$$

(b) The molecular weight of SO_2 = 64.06 g/mole so the pollutant is presumed to be sulfur dioxide.

PROBLEM 2.6. (a)

$$M = \frac{1.97 \ g \times 0.08205 \ \ell \ atm \ °K^{-1} \ mole^{-1} \times 273.15 \ °K}{1 \ atm \times 1 \ \ell} = 44.15 \ \text{g/mole}$$

(b) $\mu = \sqrt{\dfrac{3 \ P \ V}{n \ m}}$; n = moles x N (Avogadros' number) $= \dfrac{1.97}{44.15} \times 6.02 \times 10^{23}$

$= 0.27 \times 10^{23}$ molecule

The mass of a molecule is m $= \dfrac{M}{N} = \dfrac{44.15 \ g/mole}{6.02 \times 10^{23} \ molecules/mole}$

$= 7.3 \times 10^{-23}$ g/molecule

$$\mu = \sqrt{\frac{3 \times 1.01325 \times 10^6 \ dyne \ cm^{-2} \times 10^3 \ cm^3}{(0.27 \times 10^{23})(7.3 \times 10^{-23})}} = 3.9 \times 10^4 \ \text{cm/sec}$$

(c) $\mu = \sqrt{\dfrac{3P}{\rho}}$; $(3.9 \times 10^4)^2 = \dfrac{3 \times 1.01325 \times 10^6 \ dyne \ cm^{-2}}{\rho}$

$\rho = 2 \times 10^{-3}$ g/cm³

PROBLEM 2.7. (a) $P_2 = \dfrac{P_1 \ T_1}{T_1}$

in which the temperatures are given in Kelvin degrees.

$$P_2 = \frac{(30 + 14.7) \ psi \times (26 + 273.15) \ °K}{(10 + 273.15) \ °K} = 47.23 \ \ psi$$

and the gauge pressure is 47.23 − 14.7 = 32.5 psig.

(b) Keeping our eyes on the Physical Constants on the inside cover of Physical Pharmacy and on Table 1-3, and referring to a table of conversion factors in a handbook, we proceed as follows to change lb/in² into Pascals:

$$\frac{14.69594 \ lb \ (avoirdupois)}{in^2} \times \frac{453.59237 \ g}{1 \ lb \ (av)} \times \frac{in^2}{0.00064516 \ m^2}$$

$= 10332268$ g/m²

This cannot be the correct answer because in Table 1 − 3 we see that the Pascal has the units of kg m^{-1} sec^{-2}. It must be remembered that gram is a mass unit whereas pressure is a force. Thus we must multiply the mass by the acceleration of gravity 980.665 cm/sec² or for our purposes 9.80665 m sec^{-2}.

10332268 g m^{-2} x 9.80665 m sec^{-2} = 101324936 x $\dfrac{g \times m}{m^2 \times sec^2}$ x $\dfrac{1\ kg}{1000\ g}$

= 101325 kg m^{-1} sec^{-2}

In which the units kg m^{-1} sec^{-2} are found in Table 1-3 to be equivalent to Newton/meter^2 or N m^{-2}; and N m^{-2} is also called the Pascal (Pa). Thus, 1 atm = 14.69594 lb/in^2 = 101325 kg m^{-1} sec^{-2} = 101325 Pa as seen under Physical Constants on the inside cover of the book.

PROBLEM 2.8. (a) $P = \dfrac{n\,R\,T}{V} =$

$$\dfrac{0.0249\ mole \times 0.08205\ \ell\ atm\ mole^{-1}\ °K^{-1} \times 293.15\ °K}{2.37\ \ell - 0.028\ \ell\ (mouse\ volume)} = 0.256\ atm$$

Since 1 atm = 760 mm Hg = 760 torr, p = 194.3 torr

(b) From the van der Waals equation, $P = \dfrac{nRT}{V-nb} - \dfrac{an^2}{V^2}$

$P = \dfrac{0.0249\ mole \times 0.08205\ atm\ \ell/°K\ mole \times 293.15\ °K}{(2.37 - 0.028)\ell - (0.0249 \times 0.1022\ \ell/mole)}\ -$

$\dfrac{15.17\ (\ell^2\ atm/mole^2)\ (0.0249\ mole)^2}{(2.37 - 0.028)^2\ \ell^2} = 0.254\ atm = 193.3\ torr$

PROBLEM 2.9. (a) From the ideal gas equation, P = $\dfrac{n}{V}$ RT,

$P = \left(\dfrac{0.193\ mole}{7.35\ \ell}\right) 0.08205\ \dfrac{\ell\ atm}{deg\ mole}$ x 295.15°K = 0.636 atm

(b) Using the van der Waals equation, P = $\dfrac{n\,R\,T}{V - n\,b} - \dfrac{a\,n^2}{V^2}$

$P = \dfrac{(0.193\ mole)(0.08205\ (\ell\ atm)/(°K\ mole)(295.15\ °K)}{7.35\ \ell - 0.193\ mole\ (0.1344\ \ell/mole)}$

$- \dfrac{17.38\ (\ell^2\ atm/mole^2)\ (0.193)^2\ mole^2}{(7.35\ \ell)^2} = 0.626\ atm$

PROBLEM 2.10.

$$a = \frac{27 \, (0.08205 \, \ell \, atm/\, ^{\circ}K \, mole)^2 \, (263 + 273.15 \, ^{\circ}K)^2}{64 \times 54 \, atm} = 15.12 \, \text{liter}^2 \, \text{atm} \, \text{mole}^{-2}$$

$$b = \frac{0.08205 \, \ell \, atm/\, ^{\circ}K \, mole \, (263 + 273.15) \, ^{\circ}K}{8 \times 54 \, atm} = 0.1019 \, \text{liter/mole}$$

PROBLEM 2.11. (a) $\quad n = \dfrac{PV}{RT}$

$$= \frac{12.3 \, atm \times 0.80 \, \ell}{0.08205 \, \ell \, atm \, ^{\circ}K^{-1} \, mole^{-1} \times 298.15 \, ^{\circ}K} = 0.402 \, \text{mole}$$

0.402 mole x 44.01 g/mole = 17.69 g or 0.0177 kg of CO_2 at 25°C and 12.3 atm.

(b) When the pressure is lowered to 1 atm at 25 °C,

$$P_1V_1 = P_2V_2; \quad V_2 = \frac{12.3 \, atm \times 0.8 \, \ell}{1 \, \ell} = 9.84 \, \text{liter}$$

(c) The volume of 17.69 g at 25°C and 1 atm is

$$V = \frac{17.69 \, g}{0.001836 \, g/cm^3} = 9635 \, \text{cm}^3 = 9.64 \, \text{liter}.$$

The results, 9.84 liter from Boyle's law, and 9.64 liter from density, differs by about 2%.

PROBLEM 2.12. $\quad \ln P_2 - \ln P_1 = \dfrac{\Delta H \, (T_2 - T_1)}{R \, T_2 T_1}$

$$\ln P_2 = \frac{10,400 \, cal/mole \times 15 \, ^{\circ}K}{1.9872 \, cal \, ^{\circ}K^{-1} \, mole^{-1} \times 298.15 \, ^{\circ}K \times 313.15 \, ^{\circ}K} + 3.1697 = 4.0105$$

P_2 = 55.2 mm Hg.

PROBLEM 2.13. The equation is: $\log p = \dfrac{-\Delta H_v}{2.303 \, R} \dfrac{1}{T} + \log p_o$

Plotting log p (y axis) versus 1/T (x axis), the slope is $\dfrac{-\Delta H_v}{2.303 R}$, and the intercept,

log p_o. (Figure P2 – 1). The data needed are shown in Table P2 – 1.
The slope is calculated from two points of the graph (Figure P2 – 1):

Table P2−1 for Problem 2.13.

1/T × 10³	3.532	3.299	3.193
log p	1.3729	1.8965	2.1303

$$\text{slope} = \frac{2.170 - 1.35}{0.003175 - 0.00354}$$

$= -2.2466 \times 10^3$

$\Delta H_v = -2.303 \times 1.9872 \times (-2.2466 \times 10^3)$

$= 10{,}282$ cal/mole

The vapor pressure at 20°C is read from the graph. For $1/T = 1/(20 + 273.15)$

$= 0.00341$; log p = 1.64

p = 43.7 mm.

Using linear regression,

$\log p = -2243.448 \, \frac{1}{T} + 9.295$

$(r^2 = 0.9999)$

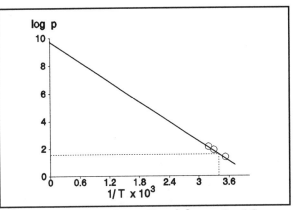

Figure P2-1 for Problem 2.13

$\Delta H_v = -(2.303) \times (1.9872) \times (-2243.448) = 10{,}267$ cal/mole.

From the equation, for T = 20°C, $\frac{1}{T} = 3.411 \times 10^{-3}$

log p = 1.643; p = 43.9 mm.

PROBLEM 2.14. (a) Between 90° and 100°C, using the Clausius−Clapeyron equation,

$$\ln p - \ln p' = \frac{\Delta H_v \, (T_2 - T_1)}{R T_1 T_2} \quad \text{and} \quad \Delta H_v = \frac{R T_1 T_2 \, (\ln p_2 - \ln p_1)}{(T_2 - T_1)} =$$

$$\frac{(1.9872) \, (373.15) \, (363.15) \, [\ln (76) - \ln (52.576)]}{(373.15 - 363.15)} = 9{,}922 \text{ cal/mole}$$

(b) Between 20° and 30°C:

$$\Delta H_v = \frac{(1.9872) \, (303.15) \, (293.15) \, [\ln (31.824) - \ln (17.535)]}{(303.15 - 293.15)}$$

$= 10{,}525$ cal/mole

Table P2 – 2 for Problem 2.14.

p (mm)	ln p	T (°K)	$1/T \times 10^3$ (°K^{-1})
6.543	1.878	278.15	3.595
9.209	2.220	283.15	3.532
17.535	2.864	293.15	3.411
31.824	3.460	303.15	3.299
525.76	6.265	363.15	2.754
760	6.633	373.15	2.680

(c) Between 5° and 10°C:

$$\Delta H_v = \frac{(1.9872)(283.15)(278.15)[\ln(9.209) - \ln(6.543)]}{(283.15 - 278.15)}$$

$\Delta H_v = 10{,}698$ cal/mole

(d) The data needed for regression over the range, 5° to 100°C are shown in Table P2 – 2

The equation is $\ln p = 20.5 - 5188.0 \dfrac{1}{T}$; ($r^2 = 0.9999$)

$\Delta H_v = (-\text{slope})(1.9872) = 5188.0 \times 1.9872 = 10310$ cal/mole (over 5° to 100°C)

The average value is 10,382 and therefore the value obtained by regression analysis, $\Delta H_v = 10{,}310$ probably also applies over the temperature range, 5° to 100°C.

PROBLEM 2.15. (a) The Clausius Clapeyron equation may be written as

$$\frac{\ln p_2}{\ln p_1} = \frac{\Delta H_v}{R}\left(\frac{1}{T_1} - \frac{1}{T_2}\right);$$ for butane:

$$\ln \frac{760}{506} = \frac{5318 \; cal/mole}{1.9872 \; cal/mole \, °K}\left\{\frac{1}{T_1} - \frac{1}{(-0.5 + 273.15)}\right\}$$

$0.000152 + 0.003667 = \dfrac{1}{T_1} = 0.003819$; $T = 261.85$ °K $= -11.30$°C

For propane:

$$\ln \frac{760}{506} = \frac{4812\ cal/mole}{1.9872\ cal\ ^\circ K\ mole^{-1}}\left\{ \frac{1}{T_1} - \frac{1}{(273.15 - 42.1)} \right\}$$

Solving for T_1, one obtains $\quad T_1 = 222.42\ ^\circ K = -50.73^\circ C$

(b) The boiling temperature of propane is well below the temperature, $-15^\circ C$, at the top of the mountain and would serve as a useful stove. On the other hand, butane has a boiling point of $-11.3^\circ C$ and would be useless for it would not vaporize and produce a flame at the mountain top temperature of $-15^\circ C$.

(c) The boiling point of water at the top of the mountain is:

$$\ln \frac{760}{506} = \frac{9717\ cal/mole}{1.9872\ cal\ ^\circ K^{-1}\ mole^{-1}}\left(\frac{1}{T_1} - \frac{1}{373.15\ ^\circ K} \right)$$

$$13.51087 = 4889.79\ \frac{1}{T_1};\quad T_1 = 361.92\ K = 88.8^\circ C.$$

The boiling point of water is $88.8^\circ C$ or 11.2° lower than $100^\circ C$, its normal boiling point (i.e., the temperature at which the vapor pressure of water is equal to the atmospheric pressure at the sea level). The water would have to be heated (boiled) an extended period of time at $88.8^\circ C$ to prepare a satisfactory cup of coffee.

PROBLEM 2.16. **(a)** Isoflurane:

$$\ln \frac{760}{p'} = \frac{6782\ cal/mole}{1.9872\ cal\ ^\circ K^{-1}\ mole^{-1}}\left\{ \frac{1}{298.15\ ^\circ K} - \frac{1}{321.65\ ^\circ K} \right\}$$

$$6.6333 - \ln p' = 0.8362;\quad p' = 329.3\ mm\ Hg$$

(b) Halothane:

$$\ln \frac{760}{243} = \frac{\Delta H_v''}{1.9872\ cal\ ^\circ K^{-1}\ mole^{-1}}\left\{ \frac{1}{293.15\ ^\circ K} - \frac{1}{323.35\ ^\circ K} \right\}$$

$$\Delta H_v'' = 7112\ cal/mole.$$

(c) See A. R. Gennaro, Ed., Remington's Pharmaceutical Sciences, Vol. 17, 1985, pp. 1041–1042.

PROBLEM 2.17. (a) Butane: $\ln \dfrac{760}{P} =$

$$\dfrac{5318\ cal/mole}{1.9872\ cal\ °K^{-1}\ mole^{-1}}\left\{\dfrac{1}{(273.15 + 40)\ °K} - \dfrac{1}{(273.15 - 0.5)\ °K}\right\}$$

$\ln 760 - \ln P = -1.2694$; $\ln P = 7.9027$; P = 2705 mm Hg = 3.56 atm.

(b) Propane: $\ln \dfrac{760}{P} =$

$$\dfrac{4811.8\ cal/mole}{1.9872\ cal\ °K^{-1}\ mole^{-1}}\left\{\dfrac{1}{(273.15+40)\ °K} - \dfrac{1}{(273.15 - 42.1)\ °K}\right\}$$

$\ln P = 6.6333 + 2.7476 = 9.3809$; P = 11860 mm Hg = 15.60 atm.

The pressures should be above 3.56 atm and 15.60 atm respectively. Note the much greater pressure required using propane because of its much lower boiling point.

(c) From your results in (a) and (b), we cannot use either plastic or aluminum containers for propane. Aluminum containers may be used for butane.

PROBLEM 2.18. (a) The pressure on the ice, P, is $= \dfrac{mass \times g}{area}$, where g is the acceleration, 981 cm/sec^2, due to gravity.

In the SI units, mass = 175 lb x 0.4536 kg/lb = 79.38 kg

The skate blade area is:

$$12\ in \times \dfrac{1}{64}\ in \times \dfrac{2.54^2\ cm^2}{in^2} \times \dfrac{1\ m^2}{100^2\ cm^2} = 1.21 \times 10^{-4}\ m^2$$

$$P = \dfrac{79.38\ kg \times 9.81\ m\ sec^{-2}}{1.21 \times 10^{-4}\ m^2} = 6.44 \times 10^6\ N\ m^{-2} = 6.44 \times 10^6\ Pa,$$

where N = newton.

$$V_\ell - V_s = \left(0.018\ \ell\ mole^{-1} \dfrac{m^3}{10^3 \ell}\right) - \left(0.01963\ \ell\ mole^{-1} \dfrac{m^3}{10^3 \ell}\right)$$

$$= -1.63 \times 10^{-6}\ m^3\ mole^{-1}$$

From the integrated form of the Clausius – Clapeyron equation,

$$\ln T - \ln(273.15) = \dfrac{(-1.63 \times 10^{-6}\ m^3\ mole^{-1})\ (6.44 \times 10^6 Pa)}{6025\ J\ mole^{-1}}$$

$\ln T = 5.6100 - 0.0017 = 5.6083$; T = 272.68 °K;

$\Delta T = 272.68 - 273.15 = -0.470°K$

(b) Using the approximation, $\frac{\Delta T}{\Delta P} = T\frac{\Delta V}{\Delta H_f}$,

$$\Delta T = \frac{273.15°K \; (-1.63 \times 10^{-6} \; m^3 \; mole^{-1})}{6025 \; J \; mole^{-1}} (6.44 \times 10^6 - 101325) \, Pa = -0.468°K$$

PROBLEM 2.19. (a) Equation (2 – 17) is written, for the transition I → II as follows:

$$\frac{\Delta T}{\Delta P} = \frac{V_{II} - V_I}{\Delta H_t}$$

where T_t is the temperature of transition, ΔH_t the heat of transition, V_{II} and V_I the molar volumes of forms II and I, respectively.

$$V_I = \frac{molecular \; weight}{density} = \frac{255.32}{1.50} = 170. \, 2 \; cm^3/mole$$

$$V_{II} = \frac{255.32}{1.55} = 164.7 \; cm^3/mole$$

$$\frac{\Delta T}{\Delta P} = (161 + 273.15) \; °K \; \frac{(164.7 - 170.2) \times 10^{-3} \, \ell}{(1420/24.22) \, \ell \; atm} = -0.041° K/atm$$

The temperature decreases when ΔP increases, thus the transition temperature is lowered.

(b) 2757.6 bar = 2757.6 x 0.987 atm/bar = 2721.75 atm

$$(-0.041 \; \frac{°K}{atm}) \times 2721.75 \; atm = -111.59°K \; ; \; 434.16 - 111.59 = 322.57°K$$

322.57 °K – 273.15 = 49.42 °C.
The transition temperature is now 49.4°C. If the temperature during the processing were greater than 50°C, form I might change to form II.

PROBLEM 2.20. The data are plotted in Figure P2 – 2. The inverse of the temperature is read on the x – axis at y = 0, 1/T = 2.7 x 10^{-3} ; T = 370 °K.

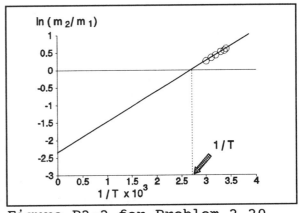

Figure P2-2 for Problem 2.20

The equation of the straight line using regression analysis is :

$$\ln \frac{m_2}{m_1} = 864.5 \frac{1}{T} - 2.34$$

For $\ln (m_2/m_1) = 0$, $864.5 \frac{1}{T} - 2.34 = 0$; and $T = 864.5/2.34 = 369.4 °K$

PROBLEM 2.21. (a)

$$\frac{70\% - 21\%}{21\% - 7\%} = \frac{49}{14} = \frac{3.5}{1}$$

Water phase (A) $= \dfrac{3.5}{3.5 + 1} = 0.78$ or 78%

Phenol phase (B) $= \dfrac{1}{3.5 + 1} = 0.22$ or 22%

For the 135 g mixture,
wt. of phase A = 0.78 x 135 = 105.3 g ≈ 105 g
wt. of phase B = 0.22 x 135 = 29.7 g ≈ 30 g

(b) The actual weight of phenol in phase A is
105 g (phase A) x 0.07 = 7.35 g and the weight of water is 105 − 7.35 = 97.65
The weight of phenol in phase B is 30 g (phase B) x 0.7 = 21 g and the weight of water is
30 − 21 = 9 g

PROBLEM 2.22. **(a)** From the plot (Figure P2 − 3), there is a single liquid phase up to 31% w/w of A present, at which point two liquid are formed (compositions are 31% w/w A and 78% w/w A). As more A is added, the amount of the second phase decreases while that of the first phase increases. When the system exceeds 78% w/w A, the two phases disappear, and the system again becomes one phase.

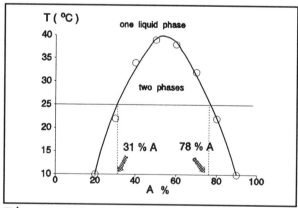

Figure P2-3 for Problem 2.22

(b) At 45°C, as shown in the plot, we are above the region of immiscibility, and hence a single phase exists for all combinations of A and B.

PROBLEM 2.23. (a) Reading off from the graph (Figure P2−4), 30% w/w A and 70% w/w B; for the conjugate phase, 80% w/w A and 20% w/w B.

(b) 20 g + 30 g = 50 g mixture. The system therefore contains 40 % A (point d in Figure P2−4) and 60 % B. The ratio,

$$\frac{A}{B} = \frac{dc}{db} = \frac{80\ \% - 40\ \%}{40\ \% - 30\ \%} = \frac{40}{10}$$

Approximately 40 g A and 10 g B

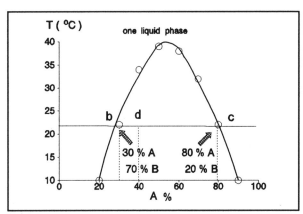

Figure P2-4 for Problem 2.23

PROBLEM 2.24. (a) From the graph (Figure P2−5), 39⁰C.

(b) If we add B, we go to the left on Figure P2−5 and at 10°C, we must go to 80% B to reach a single phase. Adding 15 g B gives 20 g B and 5 g A. This is 20/25 = 0.8 or 80% B, so 5 g of A is 20%. The answer is therefore 15 g of B added.

(c) We must go to the right on Figure P2−5 and at 10°C to 90% A before we arrive at a single phase. If we add 40 g of A to make 45 g of A and 5 g of B (we have a total of 50 g), 45/50 = 0.9 or 90% of A and therefore 10% B. The answer is 40 g of A added.

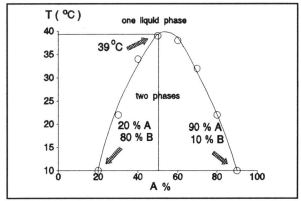

Figure P2-5 for Problem 2.24

PROBLEM 2.25. (a) Reading off from the graph (Figure P2−6), 20 % w/w A, 59 % w/w B and 21 % w/w C.

(b) $\dfrac{84 - 45}{45 - 21} = 1.625$

$100 \times \dfrac{1.625}{1 + 1.625} = 61.9$

$100 \times \dfrac{1}{1 + 1.625} = 38$

The answer is approximately 38 and 62 g.

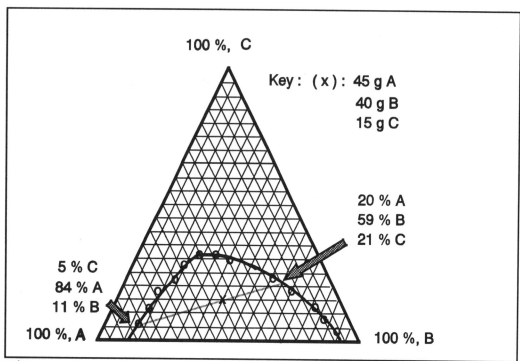

Figure P2-6 for Problems 2.25 and 2.26

PROBLEM 2.26. (a) From the graph (Figure P2−6), a single liquid phase system contains approximately 30% w/w A, 41%w/w B, and 29% w/w C when a second liquid phase separates. When the composition of the system is approximately 81% w/w A, 11% w/w B and 8% w/w C, the system reverts to one liquid phase.

(b) The solution contains 50% B, 35% A and 15% C, that is

$$0.5 \times 5 = 2.5 \text{ g B}$$
$$0.35 \times 5 = 1.75 \text{ g C}$$
$$0.15 \times 5 = 0.75 \text{ g A}.$$

The final solution is 100 g, so we need 100 − 0.5 = 95 g of solution, corresponding to 95 g of A. We had before 0.75 g of A, so the total amount of A in the final solution is

$$0.75 + 95 = 95.75 \text{ g of A}$$

Therefore, the composition is 95.75 g of A, 2.5 g of B and 1.75 g of C. This final point is not shown on Figure P2−6.

PROBLEM 2.27. (a) From the graph (Figure P2−7) we need to find the point (a single phase system) where A = 45%, B = 25% and C = 30% by adding mixture A + C. The amount of B, 40 gram, does not change. Since B is 40 g, corresponding to 25% of the mixture, the total amount of mixture is 40 x 4 = 160 g;

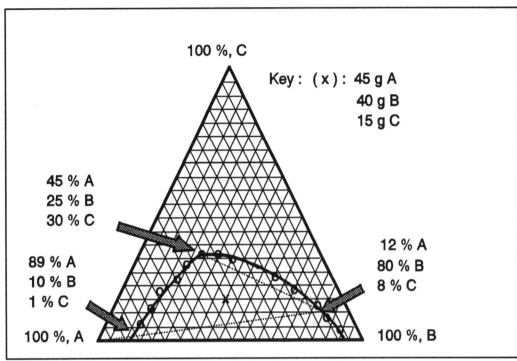

Figure P2-7 for Problem 2.27

$$160g \times 30\% = 48 \text{ g of C}$$
$$160 \text{ g} \times 45\% = 72 \text{ g of A}$$

Initially, we had 15 g of C; 48 − 15 = 33 g of C added

The amount of A added is 72 − 45 = 27 g of A

The total amount added is 33 + 27 = 60 g

(b) The composition of the one phase system is read off from the graph: A = 45%, B = 25%, C = 30%

(c) Since only B is added, A and C remain constant, A = 72 g and C = 48 g.

To get a single phase, we need 12% A, 80% B and 8% C (see Figure P2 − 7). The **total** amount of solution is calculated from the amount of A and its percent:

$$72 \times \frac{100\%}{12\%} = 600 \text{ g total solution}$$

The same result is obtained from the amount and percent of C:

$$48 \times \frac{100\%}{8\%} = 600 \text{ g total solution}$$

B is 80% of this solution corresponding to 600 x 0.8 = 480 g
We had 40 g of B, so the amount of B added is 480 − 40 = 440 g

(d) The composition is, as we read from the graph, approximately 12% A, 80% B and 8% C.

(e) Now, we add A to this solution leaving B and C at 440 g and 48 g respectively, as obtained in part (c). Reading off from the graph, Figure P2−7, we need 89% A, 1% C and 10% B.
The total amount of solution as calculated from the amount of B and its percent in the mixture is

$$440 \text{ g} \times \frac{100\%}{10\%} = 4400 \text{ g}$$

The amount of C is 48 g x $\frac{100\%}{1\%}$ = 4800 g

They should be equivalent; the difference is due to difficulties in reading off accurately from the graph. We take an average, and the total amount is $\frac{4400+4800}{2}$ = 4600 g

The amount of A needed is 4600 x 0.89 = 4094 g. Since we had 72 g of A (see part c), the amount of A added is 4094 − 72 = 4022 g

(f) Reading from the graph, 89% w/w A, 10% B and 1% w/w C (approximately).

CHAPTER 3
Thermodynamics

PROBLEM 3.1. Temperature is most frequently measured using thermometers; what we actually observe is the volume change, or the change in the height of a liquid in a capillary.

Temperature is proportional to the change of volume, and it is easier to measure in a liquid. We need the substance to be a liquid at the temperature at which we wish to measure it. Alcohol is a liquid even at very low temperatures (melting point = $-117.3°C$) so it is appropriate for the measurement of low temperatures. Its boiling point is relatively low, $78°C$ and it is not well suited to the measurement of high temperatures on the earth.

Mercury has a higher boiling point ($356.6°C$) and allows one to measure high temperatures, however its melting point is higher than that of alcohol (m.p. = $-38.87°C$), so temperatures below $-38.87°C$ cannot be measured using mercury in a capillary tube.

PROBLEM 3.2. Volume of the vapor:

$$V_{(gas)} = \frac{nRT}{P} = \frac{1.73\ mole \times 0.0821\ \ell\ atm\ °K^{-1}\ mole^{-1} \times 373\ °K}{0.68\ atm} = 77.91\ \text{liter}$$

Volume of the liquid at 373 °K:

18.795 ml/mole = 0.018795 liter/mole

1.73 mole x 0.018795 liter/mole = 0.0325 liter

W = $P\Delta V$ = 0.68 atm x (77.91 − 0.033) liter = 52.96 liter atm.

52.96 liter atm x 101.328 J/(liter atm) = 5366 J

PROBLEM 3.3.   200 kg of water requires (200 x 10^3 gram) x 1 cal/(gram x deg) = 200 x 10^3 cal/deg

$$\Delta T = \frac{3600 \times 10^3\ cal}{200 \times 10^3\ cal/degree} = 18°K = 18°C$$

The final temperature is 25 + 18 = 43°C.

PROBLEM 3.4. (a) 1 lb (av) = 453.59 gram/lb x 80 lb = 36287.2 gram

Work = m g h = (36287.2 gram)(981 cm s^{-2})(61 cm) = 2.17 x 10^9 gram cm^2 s^{-2}

= 2.17 x 10^9 erg;   (2.17 x 10^9) erg x 1 J/10^7 erg = 217.15 J per lift

(217.15 J/lift)(500 lifts) = 108575 J

$$\frac{108575\ J}{4.184\ J/cal} = 25950\ \text{cal} = 26\ \text{kcal (food calories)}$$

(b) $\dfrac{26\ kcal}{9\ kcal/gram}$ = 2.9 gram; $\dfrac{2.9\ gram}{454\ gram/lb}$ = 0.006 lb

(c) $\dfrac{500 \ lifts}{0.006 \ lb} = \dfrac{x \ lifts}{1 \ lb}$; x = 8333 lifts

(d) Thus it becomes quite clear that although exercise such as weight lifting is excellent to tone the muscles of the body and keep them functionating properly, it contributes very little to weight reduction in a diet regimen. Over 8000 lifts of the 80 lb weight would actually be required to lose 1 pound of fat from the body!

PROBLEM 3.5. $\quad \dfrac{3000 \ kcal}{10.0 \ kcal/mole} = 300$ mole

1 mole of water weights 18.015 gram; 300 x 18.015 gram/mole = 5404.5 gram. Since the density of water at 25°C is 0.997047 gram/cm³,

$$\frac{5404.5 \ gram}{0.997047 \ gram \ cm^{-3}} = 5420.5 \ cm^3 \text{ or } 5.4 \text{ liters per day.}$$

PROBLEM 3.6. The change in potential energy of the mass of water, m, as it falls through a height h is mgh. The heat or thermal energy Q created by this weight of fall is $C \Delta T$ per kilogram or $mC \Delta T$ for a mass of m kg. The formula for the specific heat C (the heat to raise 1 kg of material by 1°C or 1 °K) is

$$C = \frac{Q}{m \ \Delta T} \text{ and } Q = m \ C \ \Delta T$$

The potential energy resulting from the height, h = 280.42 meter, of the falls is converted into kinetic energy or heat of friction of the falling water Q, and we can write

$$m \ g \ h = m \ C \ \Delta T \quad \text{and} \quad \Delta T = \frac{g \ h}{C}$$

Notice that the mass m cancels so we need not consider the mass of water constituting the falls. Using SI units we obtain:

$$C = 1 \text{ cal gram}^{-1} \ ^{\circ}K^{-1} \times \frac{4.184 \ J}{cal} \times \frac{10^3 \ gram}{kg} \ ^{\circ}K^{-1} = 4.184 \times 10^3 \ J \ kg^{-1} \ ^{\circ}K^{-1}$$

$$\Delta T = \frac{9.8 \ m \ s^{-2} \times 280.42 \ m}{4.184 \times 10^3 \ J/kg \ ^{\circ}K} = 0.66 \ ^{\circ}K$$

In the cgs units,

$$C = 1 \ cal \ gram^{-1} \ ^{\circ}K^{-1} \frac{4.184 \times 10^7 erg}{1 \ cal} \ gram^{-1} \ ^{\circ}K^{-1} = 4.184 \times 10^7 \frac{erg}{gram \ ^{\circ}K}$$

$$\Delta T = \frac{980 \ cm \ s^{-2} \times 28042 \ cm}{4.184 \times 10^7 \ erg/gram \ ^{\circ}K} = 0.66°C$$

PROBLEM 3.7. First we must change °F into °C using the formula:

$$°C = \frac{5 \ (°F - 32)}{9}$$

If °F = 0, $°C = \dfrac{5 \ (0 - 32)}{9} = -17.78 \ °C$

If °F = 0.20, $°C = \dfrac{5 \ (0.20 - 32)}{9} = -17.67 \ °C$

0.2°F difference in temperature is 17.78°C − 17.67°C = 0.11°C or 0.11°K.

$h = \dfrac{C \ \Delta T}{g}$ where C is 4.184 x 10^7 erg gram^{-1} °K^{-1} in the cgs units (see problem 3.6)

$h = \dfrac{4.184 \times 10^7 \ erg \ gram^{-1} \ °K^{-1} \times 0.11°K}{981 \ cm \ sec^{-2}}$ = 4691.5 cm = 46.9 meters

$\dfrac{4691.5 \ cm}{30.48 \ cm/ft}$ = 154 ft

PROBLEM 3.8.   The heat capacity of iron is 107.4 cal/(kg°K) = 107.4 cal/(kg°K) x 4.184 J/cal = 449.4 J/(kg°K) in the SI units.

$\Delta T = \dfrac{gh}{C_v} = \dfrac{9.8 \ m/sec^2 \times 93 \ m}{449.4 \ J/kg \ °K}$ = 2.03°K or 2.03°C

PROBLEM 3.9.
$C_p(CO) = 6.342 + (1.836 \times 10^{-3} \times 298.15) - (0.2801 \times 10^{-6} \times 298.15^2) = 6.864$
$C_p(H_2) = 6.947 - (0.2 \times 10^{-3} \times 298.15) + (0.4808 \times 10^{-6} \times 298.15^2) = 6.930$
$C_p(CH_3OH) = 4.398 + (24.274 \times 10^{-3} \times 298.15) - (6.855 \times 10^{-6} \times 298.15^2) = 11.025$
The units on C_p are cal/(°K mole). For the reaction,
$\Delta C_p = 11.025 - [6.864 + (2 \times 6.930)] = -9.699$ cal/(°K mole)

PROBLEM 3.10. $\Delta H_2^° - (-21.68) = -9.699 \times 10^{-3} (308.15 - 298.15)$;

$\Delta H_2^° = -0.09699 - 21.68 = -21.78$ kcal/mole

PROBLEM 3.11. $\Delta H° = \Delta H° (Ca(OH)_2)(s) - \Delta H° (CaO)(s) + \Delta H° (H_2O)(liq.)$
$-15.6 = \Delta H° (Ca(OH)_2) - (-151.9 - 68.3)$
$\Delta H° (Ca(OH)_2) = -235.8$ kcal/mole

PROBLEM 3.12. (a) $\Delta H° = -48.10 - (-26.416 + 0) = -21.684$ kcal/mole

(b) $\Delta G° = -38.90 - (-32.78 + 0) = -6.12$ kcal/mole

$$\Delta S° = \frac{\Delta H° - \Delta G°}{T} = \frac{-21.684 - (-6.12)}{298.15} = -0.05220 \text{ kcal/(mole deg) or}$$

-52.20 cal/(mole deg)

The entropy change from the data in the table is

$\Delta S° = 56.63 - [(2 \times 31.208) + 47.219] = -53.01$ cal/(mole degree)

This value compares with that obtained above (-1.50 % difference).

PROBLEM 3.13. Efficiency $= \dfrac{T_2 - T_1}{T_2} = \dfrac{482 - 303}{482} = 0.37$ or 37%

PROBLEM 3.14. The work to discharge 79.8 cal/g x 453.6 gram = 36197 cal is

$$-W = \frac{296 - 273}{273} \times 36197 \text{ cal} = 3050 \text{ cal}$$

3050 cal x 4.184 J/cal $= 1.28 \times 10^4$ J

The coefficient of performance is

$$-\frac{W}{Q_1} = \frac{T_2 - T_1}{T_2} = \frac{296 - 273}{273} = 0.084 \text{ or } 8.4 \text{ %}$$

or $-\dfrac{W}{Q_1} = \dfrac{3050 \; cal}{36197 \; cal} = 0.084$ (8.4 %)

PROBLEM 3.15. $\Delta S = \dfrac{\Delta H_f}{T} = \dfrac{79.67 \; cal/g \times 18.02 \; g/mole}{273.15 \; °K}$

$= 5.26$ cal/mole °K

Since it is a reversible reaction,

$\Delta S_{total} = \Delta S_{H_2O} + \Delta S_{surr} = 0; \quad \Delta S_{surr} = -5.26$ cal/(mole deg)

PROBLEM 3.16. As we saw in example $3-7$ to heat the ice reversibly from $-10°C$ to $0°C$ (H_2O solid),

$H_2O(s) \rightarrow H_2O(s)$, we require the formula

$$\Delta S_1 = n \; C_p \ln\frac{T_2}{T_1} = 2 \times 9.0 \times \ln\frac{273.15}{263.15} = 0.671 \text{ cal/°K}$$

To melt ice reversibly at $0°C$, $H_2O(s) \rightarrow H_2O(liq)$,

$$\Delta S_2 = n\frac{\Delta H_{fusion}}{T} = (2\ mole) \times \frac{1437\ cal/mole}{273.15°K} = 10.52\ cal/°K$$

These 2 moles of liquid are now heated to 0.496°C,

$$H_2O\ (liq)\ (0°C) \rightarrow H_2O\ (liq)(0.496°C)$$

$$\Delta S_3 = (2\ mole)(18\ cal/°Kmole) \times \ln\frac{(273.15+0.496)°K}{273.15°K} = 0.0653\ cal/°K$$

Finally the 8.75 moles of liquid water at 20°C is cooled reversibly to 0.496°C

$$H_2O\ (liq)(20°) \rightarrow H_2O\ (liq)(0°)$$

$$\Delta S_4 = (8.75)(18) \times \left(\ln\frac{273.65}{293.15}\right) = -10.84\ cal/°K$$

The total entropy change ΔS is:

$$\Delta S = 0.671 + 10.52 + 0.0653 - 10.84 = 0.42\ cal/°K$$

The total entropy change for ice as well as for its environment, the water in the jug, is positive. The process, the melting of ice and the elevation of the temperature of the mixture slightly above zero degrees, is therefore spontaneous. It corresponds to what we would expect to happen in a thermos jug. If we allow sufficient time the temperature will gradually rise to that of the surroundings since a thermos jug is not perfectly adiabatic but rather allows the heat of the surroundings to enter the jug.

PROBLEM 3.17. $\Delta G = \Delta H - T\Delta S$; since $\Delta G = 0$,

$$\Delta S = \frac{\Delta H}{T} = \frac{29,288\ J/mole}{323.15\ °K} = 90.6\ J\ °K^{-1}\ mole^{-1}$$

PROBLEM 3.18. $\Delta G = nRT\ \ln\frac{c_2}{c_1}$, where c_2 and c_1 are the molar concentrations of

HCl; $n\Delta G = (1.9872)(310.15)\ \ln\left(\frac{0.14}{5 \times 10^{-8}}\right) = 9150\ cal/mole$

PROBLEM 3.19. $\Delta H_v = 9800\ cal/mole = 9800 \times 4.184\ J/mole = 41003\ J/mole$

$P_2 = 78\ cm\ Hg = 780\ mm = \frac{780}{760}\ atm \times 101,325\ (N\ m^{-2})/atm =$

$103991.4\ N/m^2 = 103991\ Pa$

$$\ln\frac{103991}{P_1} = \frac{41003\ J\ mole^{-1}}{8.3143\ J\ °K^{-1}\ mole^{-1}}\left(\frac{373.15 - 368.15}{368.15 \times 373.15}\right)°K^{-1}$$

$\ln P_1 = 11.5521 - 0.1795 = 11.3726;\ P_1 = 86908\ Pa$

PROBLEM 3.20. $\Delta G° = -88.99 - (-95.48) = 6.49$ kcal/mole

$$\ln K = -\frac{\Delta G°}{RT} = -\frac{6490\,cal/mole}{1.9872 \times 298.15} = -10.9539; \quad K = 1.75 \times 10^{-5}$$

PROBLEM 3.21. $\Delta G° = -140.3 - (-94.254 - 56.687) = 10.641$ kcal/mole

$\Delta H° = -164.8 - (-94.051 - 68.315) = -2.434$ kcal/ mole

Although $\Delta H°$ is negative, the process is not spontaneous because $\Delta G°$ is positive

$$\Delta S° = \frac{\Delta H° - \Delta G°}{298.15} = \frac{-2.434 - 10.641}{298.15} = -0.0439 \text{ kcal/(°K mole)}$$

$= -44$ cal/(°K mole)

The entropy change is negative, so the process is not spontaneous. The equilibrium constant is calculated from $\Delta G° = -RT \ln K$

$$\ln K = -\frac{10,641\,cal}{1.9872 \times 298.15} = -17.9600; \quad K = 1.59 \times 10^{-8}$$

PROBLEM 3.22. $\Delta H° = -26.416 + (-68.315) - (-94.051) - 0$

$= -0.68$ kcal/mole or -680 cal/mole

$\Delta S° = 47.2 + 18.5 - (51.06) - (31.208) = -16.568$ cal/deg mole

$$\ln K = \frac{\Delta S°}{R} - \frac{\Delta H°}{RT} = \frac{-16.568}{1.9872} - \frac{-680}{(1.9872)(298.15)} = -7.1896$$

$K = \exp(-7.1896) = 7.54 \times 10^{-4}$

$\Delta G° = -RT \ln K = -(1.9872)(298.15)(-7.1896) = 4260$ cal/mole

PROBLEM 3.23. (a) $\Delta G° = -113.32 - 140.29 - (-190.53 - 56.69) = -6.39$ kcal/mole

$$\ln K = \frac{-\Delta G°}{RT} = \frac{6390}{1.9872 \times 310.15} = 10.3678; \quad K = 3.20 \times 10^{4}$$

(b) $\Delta G° = -273.90 - (-190.53 - 88.99) = 5.62$ kcal/mole

$$\ln K = -\frac{5620}{1.9872 \times 310.15} = -9.1185; \quad K = 1.1 \times 10^{-4}$$

PROBLEM 3.24. (a)

$$K = \frac{[HI]^2}{[H_2][I_2]} = \frac{(1.687 \times 10^{-2})^2}{(3.84 \times 10^{-3})(1.524 \times 10^{-3})} = 48.62$$

$$K = \frac{(1.181 \times 10^{-2})^2}{(1.696 \times 10^{-3})(1.696 \times 10^{-3})} = 48.49$$

$$K = \frac{(1.270 \times 10^{-2})^2}{(5.617 \times 10^{-3})(0.5936 \times 10^{-3})} = 48.37 \; ; \; \bar{K} = \frac{\sum K}{3} = 48.49$$

(b) $\quad \ln\dfrac{48.49}{60.80} = \dfrac{\Delta H^\circ}{1.9872}\left\{\dfrac{730.75 - 666.8}{730.75 \times 666.8}\right\}.$ Solving for ΔH°, one obtains

$\Delta H^\circ = -3425$ cal or $-3425 \times 4.184 = -14330$ J.

(c) K_2 (730.75°K) is 48.49, and K_1 (666.75°K) is 60.80, therefore the equilibrium constant decreases as the temperature is raised. It indicates that the production of hydrogen iodide from its elements decreases with temperature. This does not allow us to state that the reaction is exothermic, because the equilibrium constant is related to the free energy, which is composed of two terms: enthalpy and entropy. The free energy change, as calculated from the equilibrium constants, is negative and it could be due to either a negative enthalpy change (exothermic process) or to a positive favorable entropy change.

The quantitative result which allows us to state whether the reaction is exothermic is the negative enthalpy change as calculated in part **(b)**, by the use of the van't Hoff equation.

PROBLEM 3.25. At 763.8 °K, $\Delta G^\circ = -1.9872 \times 763.8 \times \ln 45.62 = -5799$ cal
By the same kind of calculations at the second and third temperatures, we obtain
$\Delta G^\circ = -5637$ and -5443 cal at 730.8 °K and 666.8 °K, respectively.

PROBLEM 3.26. (a) The data needed for the plot and for the calculation of the regression line are found in Table P3 − 1. The vaporization and sublimation curves are shown in Figure P3 − 1.

(b) For sublimation,

$\ln P = -6146.5 \; \dfrac{1}{T} + 24.025;$

$r^2 = 0.9999$
Between −50° and 0°C,
$\Delta H_s = 1.9872 \times 6146.5$
$= 12{,}214$ cal/mole

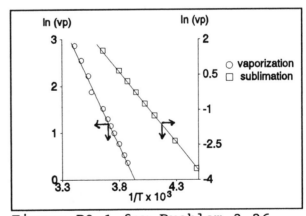

Figure P3−1 for Problem 3.26

Problem Solving: Physical Pharmacy

Table P3 – 1 for Problem 3.26.

Ice → water vapor		liquid water → water vapor	
$1/T \times 10^3$ (x)	ln (vp) (y)	$1/T \times 10^3$ (x)	ln (v p) (y)
4.481	-3.5200	3.874	0.3619
4.289	-2.3372	3.844	0.5253
4.113	-1.2521	3.800	0.7650
4.030	-0.7423	3.757	0.9988
3.950	-0.2536	3.729	1.1515
3.874	0.2159	3.702	1.3010
3.800	0.6678	3.661	1.5215
3.729	1.1029	3.595	1.8784
3.661	1.5215	3.532	2.2202
–	–	3.470	2.5485
–	–	3.411	2.8642

For vaporization,

$$\ln P = -5409 \frac{1}{T} + 21.321; r^2 = 0.9999$$

Between $-15°$ and $20°C$,

$\Delta H_v = 1.9872 \times 5409 = 10{,}749$ cal/mole

(c) $\Delta H_f = \Delta H_s - \Delta H_v = 12{,}214 - 10{,}749 = 1{,}465$ cal/mole

The experimental value is 1440 cal/mole

PROBLEM 3.27.

$$\ln K = -\frac{\Delta G°}{RT} = \frac{1727\, cal/mole}{1.9872\, cal/°K\, mole \times 298.15\, °K} = 2.912; K = 18.45$$

CHAPTER 4
Physical Properties of Drug Molecules

PROBLEM 4.1. $\bar{\nu} = \dfrac{E}{h\,c}$;

$E = hc\,\bar{\nu} = 6.626 \times 10^{-34}\,(3 \times 10^8) \times \dfrac{1}{6.780 \times 10^{-7}} = 2.93 \times 10^{-19}$ J

PROBLEM 4.2. For example, Lange's Handbook (J. A. Dean, Ed., Lange's Handbook of Chemistry, Mc Graw-Hill, New York, 1979) indicates that the sensitivity of the emission method for selenium (Se) is at 3 ppm, which is much higher than its normal whole blood level of approximately 0.1 ppm. Thus, lack of sensitivity is one of its drawbacks. Can you suggest others?

PROBLEM 4.3. (CS) = 0.02458 (EI) + 0.02718; r^2 = 0.9979.
Substituting the EI value of the urine sample in the equation gives:
CS(urine sample) = (0.02458 x 32) + 0.02718 = 0.813 μg/ml.
The amount in the 980 ml volume is 980 ml x 0.813 μg/ml = 797 μg per 24 hour sample.

PROBLEM 4.4. $c = \dfrac{A}{b \times \epsilon} = \dfrac{0.438}{1 \times 29,200} = 1.5 \times 10^{-5}$ mole/liter

$c = 1.5 \times 10^{-5}$ mole/liter x 0.1 liter x 399.4 g/mole x 1000 mg/g = 0.6 mg/tablet.

PROBLEM 4.5. $c = \dfrac{A}{b \times \epsilon}$

At 285 nm, $c = \dfrac{0.002}{1 \times 775} = 2.6 \times 10^{-6}$ mole/liter

At 276 nm, $c = \dfrac{0.002}{1 \times 951} = 2.1 \times 10^{-6}$ mole/liter

At 226 nm, $c = \dfrac{0.002}{1 \times 8570} = 2.3 \times 10^{-7}$ mole/liter. For 1/4 grain tablet = 16.2 mg of

sodium saccharin, the final concentration is

$\dfrac{0.0162\ g}{205.16\ g/mole} = 7.896 \times 10^{-5}$ mole/50 ml ;

$\dfrac{7.896 \times 10^{-5}\ mole}{50\ ml} \times \dfrac{1000\ ml}{1\ \ell} = 1.58 \times 10^{-3}$ mole/liter.

The molar concentration is larger than the minimum detectable amount at 285, 276 and 226 nm, so that any of these wavelengths are suitable for the analysis.

PROBLEM 4.6.

The concentration is $\dfrac{A}{\epsilon b} = \dfrac{0.340}{(13500)(1)} = 2.52 \times 10^{-5}$ M

2.52×10^{-5} mole/liter x 151.2 g/mole = 3.8×10^{-3} g/liter = 3.8×10^{-3} mg/ml.

The amount of acetaminophen in the 400 mg portion assayed, corresponding to the weight of one tablet) is:

3.8×10^{-3} mg/ml x (250 x 250) ml = 237.5 mg per tablet.

The deviation from the labeled amount is

$\dfrac{250 - 237.5}{250} \times 100 = 5\%$

The deviation is within the limits established.

PROBLEM 4.7. Such a curve would be produced where the change in absorbance to change in concentration decreases as the concentration increases. In reality, such a curve is often seen for Beer's law plots at high concentrations, due to deviations from the ideal solution behavior assumed in Beer's law. From a molecular point of view, the cause of deviations from ideal solution behavior at high concentrations can be due to solute – solute interactions such as dipole – dipole and acid – base (Lewis) interactions.

PROBLEM 4.8. $P_i = \dfrac{\epsilon - 1}{\epsilon + 2}\dfrac{M}{\rho} = \dfrac{4.34 - 1}{4.34 + 2} \times \dfrac{74.12}{0.7134} = 54.73$ cm^3/mole

$\alpha_p = \dfrac{3\,P_i}{4\,\pi\,N} = \dfrac{3 \times 54.73}{4 \times 3.1416 \times 6.02 \times 10^{23}} = 2.17 \times 10^{-23}$ cm^3

PROBLEM 4.9. For the first set:

$c = \dfrac{0.394\ mg/ml}{(281.3\ g/mole) \times (1000\ mg/g)}$

$= 1.4 \times 10^{-6}$ mole/liter

$\epsilon = \dfrac{A}{b\,c}$

$= \dfrac{0.06}{(1\ cm)(1.4 \times 10^{-6})\ mole/\ell}$

$= 4.29 \times 10^4$ liter/(mole cm)

The same kind of calculations give 4.33×10^4 and 4.25×10^4 liter mole^{-1} cm^{-1} for the second and third sets, respectively. The mean

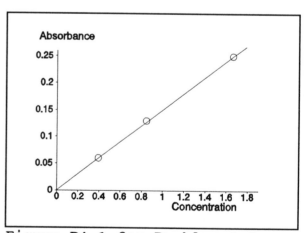

Figure P4-1 for Problem 4.9

value is $\epsilon = 4.29 \times 10^4$ liter mole^{-1} cm^{-1}. The Beer law is showed in Figure P4 – 1.

PROBLEM 4.10. $\epsilon = (182)\left(\dfrac{100\ ml}{g}\right)\left(\dfrac{1\ell}{1000ml}\right)(357.8/mole)$

= 6512 liter/(mole cm)

PROBLEM 4.11. (a) $\Delta E = \mu_H\, H\, \dfrac{1 - \sigma}{I}$

$= (1.41062 \times 10^{-26}) \times 1\ \text{tesla}\ \dfrac{1 - (-2.2 \times 10^{-6})}{1/2} = 2.8212462 \times 10^{-26}\ \text{J}$

$\nu_R = \dfrac{\Delta E}{h} = \dfrac{2.8212462 \times 10^{-26}}{6.626196 \times 10^{-34}} = 4.257716 \times 10^{7}\ \text{Hz}$

(b) $\delta = \dfrac{\Delta\nu}{\nu_R} \times 10^6 = \dfrac{(4.257716 \times 10^7) - (4.257707 \times 10^7)}{4.257707 \times 10^7} \times 10^6 = 2.11\ \text{ppm}$

PROBLEM 4.12. $\dfrac{0.80\ \mu g/ml}{60.5 - 1.2} = \dfrac{x}{38.4 - 1.2}$; $x = 0.50\ \mu g/ml$

PROBLEM 4.13. $\{\alpha\}_D^{25°} = \dfrac{\alpha\ v}{\ell\ g} = \dfrac{20° \times 100\ cm^3}{1dm \times 15.3g} = 131°$

(Actually (deg cm^3)/(dm g) or deg/(dm ρ) where ρ is the density).

PROBLEM 4.14. $P = \dfrac{\epsilon - 1}{\epsilon + 2}\ \dfrac{M}{\rho} = \dfrac{78.5 - 1}{78.5 + 2} \times \dfrac{18.015}{0.997} = 17.4\ cm^3/mole$

PROBLEM 4.15. The absence of a strong band between $1600 - 2000\ cm^{-1}$ excludes cocaine since this should be the region for strong carbonyl absorption, while the bands at $1400 - 1500\ cm^{-1}$ (aromatic) could be for either compound, and the $3200 - 3700\ cm^{-1}$ (hydroxyl) band indicates codeine.

PROBLEM 4.16. From equation (4 – 22),

$C = \dfrac{W}{V} \times \dfrac{I_u}{I_s} \times \dfrac{EW_u}{EW_s} = 25\ \dfrac{mg}{1\ capsule} \times \dfrac{1200}{7059} \times \dfrac{291.9/6}{74.1/9} = 25\ \text{mg per capsule}$

PROBLEM 4.17.   The protons of water give a signal whereas deuterium has no spin and produces no interfering signal. Deuterated chloroform or deuterated methanol would also be suitable solvents.

PROBLEM 4.18. (a) From Table 4-1,

R_m = 2.418 + (4 x 1.100) + 1.525 = 8.343 cm³/mole.

From equation 4-24:

$$R_m = \frac{n^2 - 1}{n^2 + 2} \frac{M}{\rho} = \left[\frac{(1.326)^2 - 1}{(1.326)^2 + 2}\right] \frac{32.04}{0.7866} = 8.218$$

(b) The units on R_m are $\dfrac{g/mole}{g/cm^3}$ = cm³/mole

PROBLEM 4.19. $[\Theta] = \dfrac{[\Psi]\ M}{100} = \dfrac{1.04 \times 10^5 \times 350}{100} =$

$3.64 \times 10^5 \dfrac{deg/ml}{mole\ dm} \times \dfrac{1\ell}{1000\ ml} = 364$ liter/(mole dm)

PROBLEM 4.20. $n = \dfrac{\sin(i)}{\sin(r)} = \dfrac{\sin(45°)}{\sin(r)} = 1.627$

$\sin(r) = \dfrac{\sin(45°)}{1.627} = \dfrac{0.7071}{1.627} = 0.4346;\quad r = 25°\ 45'$

PROBLEM 4.21. $\{\alpha\}_D^{20} = \dfrac{\alpha\ v}{\ell\ g} = \dfrac{15.2 \times 10}{1 \times g} = 30.4$

g = 152/30.4 = 5 g in 10 ml ; the concentration of digoxin is 0.5 g/ml.

CHAPTER 5
Solutions of Nonelectrolytes

PROBLEM 5.1. (a) weight percent $= \dfrac{0.5}{100.5} \times 100 = 0.498\%$

(b) Molal concentration:

$\dfrac{0.5g}{342\ g/mole} = 0.00146$ mole/(100 g) $= 0.0146$ mole/(kg water)

(c) Mole fraction:

100 g of H_2O corresponds to $\dfrac{100\ g}{18.01528\ g/mole} = 5.55084$ moles; from the calculations

above, moles of sucrose per 100 g of $H_2O = 0.00146$. The mole fraction of sucrose is:

$X_2 = \dfrac{0.00146}{0.00146 + 5.55084} = 0.00026$

Mole fraction of water: $\quad X_1 = (1 - 0.00026) = 0.99974$

PROBLEM 5.2. Molarity:

7% w/w = 70 g/(kg water)

$\dfrac{70}{92.0473} = 0.76048$ mole/1000 g ; $\quad \dfrac{1000g}{1.0149g/ml} = 985.3188$ ml

$\dfrac{0.76048\ mole}{985.3188\ ml} = \dfrac{x}{1000\ ml}$; $\quad x = 0.7718$ M.

Molality:

1000 − 70 = 930 g H_2O

$\dfrac{0.76048}{930\ g} = \dfrac{x}{1000\ g}$; $\quad x = 0.8177$ molal

Percent by volume:

$\dfrac{7\ g}{1.2609\ g/ml} = 5.55$ ml glycerin

$\dfrac{100\ g}{1.0149\ g/ml} = 98.53$ ml solution; $\quad \dfrac{5.55}{98.53} \times 100 = 5.63\%$ by volume

PROBLEM 5.3. $\quad N_1V_1 = N_2V_2$; $\quad N \times 25 = 0.5 \times 20$; $\quad N = 0.40$

PROBLEM 5.4. Equivalent weight = $\dfrac{142}{2}$ = 71 g;

71 x 0.5 N x 1.2 liters = 42.6 g

PROBLEM 5.5. **(a)** Number of equivalents per mole:

HCl = 1; H_3PO_4 = 3; $Ba(OH)_2$ = 2

(b) Equivalent weights: HCl = 36.5/1 = 36.5 ; H_3PO_4 = 98/3 = 32.7 ; $Ba(OH)_2$ = 171.4/2 = 85.7. (The units are g/Eq).

PROBLEM 5.6. For Na^+, 242; for Al^{3+}, 242/3 = 80.7; for $(SO_4^{2-})_2$, 242/4 = 60.5 g/Eq

PROBLEM 5.7. Eq wt (g/Eq) = $\dfrac{g/\ell}{Eq/\ell}$

or Eq/liter = $\dfrac{g/\ell}{Eq\ wt}$; 3 mEq/liter = $\dfrac{mg/\ell}{mg/mEq}$

3 mEq/liter x 87 mg/mEq = 261 mg/liter

PROBLEM 5.8. $\dfrac{310\ g/mole}{6\ Eq/mole}$ = 51.667 Eq wt (g/Eq)

51.667 g = 1 Equivalent = 1 liter of 1 N solution.

51.667 x $\dfrac{0.170\ \ell}{1\ \ell}$ x $\dfrac{0.67\ N}{1\ N}$ = 5.88 g

PROBLEM 5.9. n−butane, 50 g/58.12 (g/mole) = 0.8603 mole

n−pentane, 50 g/72.15 (g/mole) = 0.6930 mole

From the Raoult law, X p° = p. For n−butane,

$p_B = X_B \cdot p_B^o = \dfrac{0.8603}{0.8603 + 0.6930}$ (2.3966) = 1.327 atm

1.327 atm x 14.70 (lb/sq in.)/atm = 19.507 lb/sq in.

For n−pentane, $p_p = \dfrac{0.6930}{0.6930 + 0.8603}$ (0.6999) = 0.312 atm

0.312 atm x 14.70 (lb/sq in.)/atm = 4.586 lb/sq in.

PROBLEM 5.10. (a) Freon 11, p_{11} = 15 x 0.6 = 9 lb/sq in.

Freon 12, p_{12} = 85 x 0.4 = 34 lb/sq in.

(b) P = Σp = 34 + 9 = 43 lb/sq in.

(c) The total vapor pressure is greater than 35 lb/sq in., therefore the aerosol cannot be safely packaged in the glass container.

PROBLEM 5.11. (a) Henry's law:

$p_{solute} = k\, X_{solute}$
Raoult's law: $p_{solvent} = p^o_{solvent}\, X_{solvent}$
Both apply to very dilute solutions. Raoult's
law apply to the solvent (when it is in high
concentration, that is in a dilute solution), and
Henry's law applies to the solute at very low
concentration.

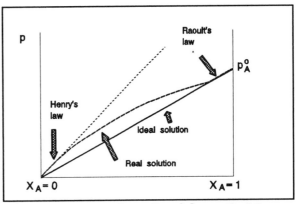

Figure P5-1 for Problem 5.11

(b) Henry's law allows one to calculate the
solubility knowing the Henry's law constant and the partial pressure of the solute. Henry's law
becomes identical to Raoult's law for an ideal solution, for which through the entire range of
concentration, $k = p^o$. Figure P5 – 1 shows an example of positive deviation from Raoult's
law: Henry's law applies when A is very dilute and Raoult's law when A is almost the pure
component.

PROBLEM 5.12. (a) $X_{O_2} = \dfrac{0.20\ atm}{4.34 \times 10^4\ atm} = 4.61 \times 10^{-6}$

$X_{N_2} = \dfrac{0.80\ atm}{8.57 \times 10^4\ atm} = 9.33 \times 10^{-6}$

(b) The total mole fraction concentration of gases in water is thus
$(4.61 \times 10^{-6}) + (9.33 \times 10^{-6}) = 13.94 \times 10^{-6}$

(c) The fraction of oxygen in water is: $\dfrac{4.61 \times 10^{-6}}{13.94 \times 10^{-6}} = 0.33 = \dfrac{1}{3}$

(d) In air, oxygen constitutes 0.20 of the total pressure or 1/5. Thus the dissolved air a fish
breathes is greater proportionately in oxygen than the air we land animals breathe.

PROBLEM 5.13. $X_{O_2} = \dfrac{P_{O_2}}{k} = \dfrac{200\ mm\ Hg}{3.3 \times 10^7\ mm\ Hg} = 6.06 \times 10^{-6}$

PROBLEM 5.14. (a) From equation (5 – 51):

$M_2 = K_f \dfrac{1000\ w_2}{\Delta T_f\, w_1} = \dfrac{1.86 \times 1000 \times 1}{0.573 \times 100} = 32.46\, g/mole$

(b) The molality is $m = \dfrac{10\ g/kg}{32.46} = 0.3081$

$\Delta T_b = K_b\, m = 0.51 \times 0.3081 = 0.157°$

The boiling point is

$100° + 0.157° = 100.157°C$

(c) $\pi = RTm = 0.0821 \times 298.15 \times 0.3081$

$= 7.54$ atm

If we apply equation (5 – 54), with ΔT_f

$= 1.86 \times 0.3081 = 0.573°C,$

$\pi = (12 \times 0.573) - (0.021 \times 0.573^2)$

$= 6.87$ atm

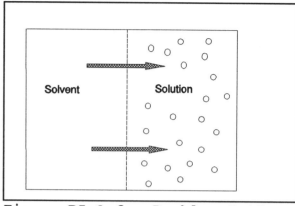

Figure P5-2 for Problem 5.15

PROBLEM 5.15. (a) From Table

5 – 4, $\Delta p = 0.43$ m, and $\pi = RTm$

$= 0.0821(25 + 273.15)m = 24.48$ m,

$\dfrac{\pi}{\Delta p} = \dfrac{24.48\ m}{0.43\ m};\quad \pi = 56.93\ \Delta p$

(b) Pure solvent has a high escaping tendency relative to the solution. See Figure P5 – 2. The solvent passes through the membrane from a region of high escaping tendency (pure solvent region) to the region of low escaping tendency (solution). The solute particles cannot pass through the semipermeable membrane; they tend to lower the chemical potential or escaping tendency on the solution side of the membrane. For a thermodynamic explanation, see Chapter 5, the section on Thermodynamics of Osmotic Pressure.

PROBLEM 5.16. From vapor pressure lowering,

$M_2 = \dfrac{w_2\, M_1\, p_1^o}{w_2\, \Delta p_1} = \dfrac{105 \times 18.015 \times 123.8}{500(123.8 - 122.6)}\ 6{,}218 = 390$ g/mole

From boiling point elevation:

$M_2 = K_b \dfrac{1000\ w_2}{w_1\ \Delta T_b} = \dfrac{0.51 \times 1000 \times 105}{500 \times 0.271} = 395$ g/mole

From osmotic pressure:

Grams of solute in 1000 g of solvent, $w_2 = 105 \times 2 = 210$ g

$M_2 = \dfrac{R\, T\, w_2}{1000\ \pi} = \dfrac{0.0821 \times 329.15 \times 210}{1000 \times 0.0138} = 411$ g/mole

PROBLEM 5.17. The data needed are shown in Table P5 – 1.

(a) By extrapolation, that is, "by eye", $\Delta H_v = 47.5$ cal/g (Figure P5 – 3).

47.5 cal/g x 153.84 g/mole = 7307.4 cal/mole at the boiling point, 76.7°C or 349.85°K

Table P5 – 1 for Problem 5.17.

ΔH_v (cal/g)	52.47	52.06	51.78	51.22	50.78	50.04
°C	– 6.67	– 1.11	4.44	15.56	21.11	26.67

Table P5 – 1 (continued)

ΔH_v (cal/g)	50.01	49.67	49.28	48.83
°C	32.22	37.78	43.33	48.89

Using this value in the equation, one obtains

$$K_b = \frac{RT_b^2 M}{1000 \, \Delta H_v}$$

$$= \frac{(1.9872)(349.85)^2(153.84)}{(1000)(7307.4)}$$

= 5.12 (deg kg)/mole

(b) Using a cubic regression of ΔH_v against temperature (data from Table 5 – 1), the equation is:

ΔH_v (cal/g) = 52.0594867
– 0.05916 t – 0.000306 t^2 + 0.00000378 t^3
(r^2 = 0.9905)

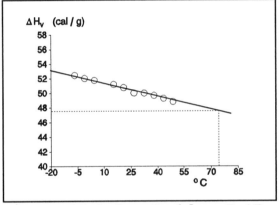

Figure P5-3 for Problem 5.17

Substituting in the equation for t = 76.7°C (boiling point),

ΔH_v = 47.4274 cal/g; 47.4274 cal x 153.84 g/mole = 7296.2 cal/mole at the boiling point,

76.7°C or 349.85°K

Using this value,

$$K_b = \frac{(1.9872)(349.85)^2(153.84)}{(1000)(7296.2)} = 5.13 \text{ (deg kg)/mole}$$

PROBLEM 5.18. $\quad \Delta T_b = K_b m; \quad m = \frac{0.28}{0.513} = 0.5458;$

grams of drug in 1 kg of solvent = 150 g;

$m = 0.5458 = \frac{150 \, g}{m.w.}; \quad$ m.w. = 275 g/mole

PROBLEM 5.19. (a)

$$\Delta T_b = \frac{R\,T_b^2}{\Delta H_v^o}\,X_2 = \frac{1.9872 \times (373.15)^2}{9720} \times 0.1239 = 3.53\,°C$$

To convert it to °F, $°F = \dfrac{9\,(°C) + 160}{5}$;

Take 100°C, °F = 212, then (100 + 3.53)°C, °F = 218.35; 218.35 − 212 = 6.35°F

(b) $m = \dfrac{1000\,X_2}{M_1\,(1 - X_2)} = \dfrac{1000 \times 0.1239}{18.0153\,(1 - 0.1239)} = 7.8501$

$\Delta T_b = K_b m = 0.51 \times 7.8501 = 4.00\,°C$ or $7.20\,°F$

PROBLEM 5.20 (a). $\Delta T_b = K_b m = 3.63 \times 0.437 = 1.586\,°C$

(b) 0.437 mole/kg H_2O × 172.2 g/mole = 75.25 g anthracene and 1000 g of water;

$$\Delta T_b = K_b \frac{1000\,w_2}{w_1\,M_2} = 3.63 \times \frac{1000 \times 75.25}{1000 \times 172.2} = 1.586°$$

PROBLEM 5.21.

$$M_2 = K_b \frac{1000\,w_2}{w_1\,\Delta T_f} = 5.12 \times \frac{1000 \times 0.2223}{1000 \times 0.00124} = 918\ g/mole$$

PROBLEM 5.22. $m = \dfrac{\Delta T_f}{K_f} = \dfrac{0.120}{1.86} = 0.06452$ mole solute/kg solvent

5 g of solute in 250 g of water = 20 g of solute in 1000 g of solvent

molality, m = 0.06452 = $\dfrac{g\ solute/1000\ g\ solvent}{m.\ w.} = \dfrac{20}{m.\ w.}$

Solving for the molecular weight, m.w. = 310 g/mole

PROBLEM 5.23. (a)   The molality of the solution is m = $\dfrac{10}{26000} = 0.0004$

The freezing point depression is $\Delta T_f = 1.86 \times 0.0004 = 0.0007\,°C$

(b)   The osmotic pressure is

$\pi = 0.0004 \times 0.0821 \times 293.15 = 0.0096$ atm

0.0096 atm × $\dfrac{760\ mm}{atm}$ × $\dfrac{13.5462\ g/cm^3}{1\ g/cm^3} = 98.8$ mm = 9.9 cm

(c) The freezing point depression is too small to read on most thermometers. You should use osmotic pressure to determine the molecular weight of methylcellulose.

PROBLEM 5.24. (a) Benzene

$$K_f = \frac{R\,T_f^2\,M_1}{1000\,\Delta H_f} = \frac{(1.9872)(278.65)^2(78.11)}{1000 \times 2360} = 5.10 \; deg\;kg/mole$$

(b) Phenol

$$K_b = \frac{R\,T_b^2\,M_1}{1000\,\Delta H_v} = \frac{(1.9872)(454.6)^2(94.11)}{1000 \times 9730} = 3.97 \; deg\;kg/mole$$

PROBLEM 5.25. $0.2\% = 2$ g in 1 liter solution and $\dfrac{2g}{180g/mole} = 0.0111$ M

Assuming that M = m, $\Delta T_f = 0.0111 \times 1.86 = 0.02°$

PROBLEM 5.26. $-20°F = [\dfrac{5(-20-32)}{9}]\;°C = -28.9\;°C$

$\Delta T_f = K_f m; \; m = \dfrac{28.9}{1.86} = 15.54$ molal

15.54 mole/kg x 62.07 g/mole = 964.6 g/kg water
We need about 96.6 g ethylene glycol per 100 g of fluid.

PROBLEM 5.27. (a) 5 pounds x 0.4536 kg/pound = 2.268 kg or 2268 g of sugar.
12 qt x 0.9463 liter/qt = 11.36 liter ≈ 11.36 kg = 11360 g of water

$$\Delta T_f = 1.86 \times \frac{1000 \times 2268}{11360 \times 342} = 1.09°\;C$$

The temperature can drop by only 1.09°C before the fluid freezes, therefore sucrose would not help.
(b) We would need to add a solute of smaller molecular weight to get a higher depression of the freezing point, because ΔT_f is related to the inverse of molecular weight. Thus, using the same amount in grams of methanol i.e. 2268 g (m. wt. = 32.04), one gets a larger depression of freezing point, $\Delta T_f = 11.60°C$. Do any of your students suggest that the water be drained out of the radiator overnight and refilled in the morning before driving into town?

PROBLEM 5.28. 0.3 g/60 (g/mole) = 0.005 moles/0.05 liters;

$$\pi = \frac{nRT}{V} = \frac{(0.005)(0.0821)(293.15)}{0.05} = 2.4 \text{ atm}$$

PROBLEM 5.29. **(a)** $\pi = mRT = 0.6 \times 0.0821 \times 293.15 = 14.4$ atm

(b) $\pi = \dfrac{RT}{V} \ln\dfrac{p^{\circ}}{p} = \dfrac{0.0821 \times 293.15}{0.018} \ln\left(\dfrac{17.535}{17.349}\right) = 14.3$ atm

PROBLEM 5.30. **(a)** $m = \dfrac{\Delta T_f}{K_f} = \dfrac{0.52}{1.86} = 0.2796$

$\pi = mRT = 0.2796 \times 0.0821 \times 298.15 = 6.84$ atm

(b) $X_2 = \dfrac{0.2796}{0.2796 + \dfrac{1000}{18.01534}} = 0.00501$

The vapor pressure of water at 25°C is 23.756 mm

$\Delta p = 23.756 \times 0.00501 = 0.12$ mm

Using the approximate equation,

$\Delta p = 0.018 m p_o = 0.018 \times 0.2796 \times 23.756 = 0.12$ mm Hg

PROBLEM 5.31. $M = \dfrac{c_g RT}{\pi} =$

$\dfrac{0.473 \times (1000ml/500ml) \times 0.0821 \times 298.15}{0.060} = 386 \ g/mole$

PROBLEM 5.32. **(a)** Using equation (5 – 57), $\pi = RT \dfrac{\Delta T_f}{K_f}$

$\pi = \left(0.0821\dfrac{l \ atm}{deg \ mole}\right)(273.15 \ deg)\left(\dfrac{0.198 \ deg}{1.86 \ deg \ kg \ mole^{-1}}\right) = 2.39$ atm

In a relatively diluted solution (2g/100 ml) we assume 1 liter of solution is roughly equal to 1 kg of solvent. Then all units except atmospheres cancel in the above equation.

(b) To calculate the molecular weight, M, we use the equation (5 – 56):

$\pi = \dfrac{c_g RT}{M}$ in which $c_g = 20$ g/liter

$2.39 \text{ atm} = \dfrac{(20g/l)(0.0821 \ l \ atm)(273.15 \ ^{\circ})}{M}$; $M = 188$ g/mole

PROBLEM 5.33. One % or 1 gram in 100 ml of solution = 10 grams per 1015 g of solution. Therefore the solution contains 10 g of drug and 1005 g of water. Using osmotic pressure:

$$\pi = RT\frac{1000\ w_2}{w_1} \times \frac{1}{M_2} = 0.0821 \times 293.15 \times \frac{1000 \times 10}{1005} \times \frac{1}{10000}$$

$$= 0.024\ \text{atm} = 0.024 \times 760 = 18.24\ \text{mm Hg};$$

$$18.24 \times \frac{13.546}{1.015} = 243\ \text{mm solution}.$$

Using boiling point elevation:

$$\Delta T_b = K_b m = K_b \frac{1000\ w_2}{w_1\ M_2} = \frac{0.51 \times 1000 \times 10}{(1015 - 10) \times 10000} = 5.07 \times 10^{-4}\ deg$$

Using freezing point depression:

$$\Delta T_f = K_f \frac{1000\ w_2}{w_1\ M_2} = \frac{1.86 \times 1000 \times 10}{1005 \times 10000} = 1.85 \times 10^{-3}\ deg$$

Using vapor pressure:

$$\Delta p = p_1^{\circ} \times \frac{w_2/M_2}{w_1/M_1} = \frac{17.54}{760} \times \frac{10/1000}{1005/18.02} = 4.14 \times 10^{-6}\ \text{atm}$$

$$= 3.14 \times 10^{-3}\ \text{mm Hg}$$

The best colligative property is osmotic pressure, because 243.2 mm of solution is easy to measure, whereas 5.07×10^{-4} deg, 1.85×10^{-3} deg and 3.14×10^{-3} mm Hg cannot be measured accurately.

CHAPTER 6
Solutions of Electrolytes

PROBLEM 6.1. $\Lambda_{\text{Na sulf}} + \Lambda_{\text{HCl}} - \Lambda_{\text{NaCl}} = \Lambda_{\text{acid}}$
$100.3 + 426.16 - 126.45 = 400$ mho cm^2/Eq

PROBLEM 6.2. $\Lambda_{o(\text{HCl})} + \Lambda_{o(\text{NaAc})} - \Lambda_{o(\text{NaCl})} = \Lambda_{o(\text{HAc})}$
$426.16 + 91.0 - 126.45 = 390.7$ mho cm^2/Eq

PROBLEM 6.3. (a) The data (Table P6 − 1) are plotted in Figure P6 − 1. The equation of the line is:

$\Lambda_c = 126.45 - 43.70 \sqrt{c}$; $r^2 = 0.9999$

Λ_o is the intercept, 126.45 ohm^{-1} cm^2/Eq (ohm^{-1} = mho).

(b) From the definition of transference number and the Kohlrausch equation (6 − 23), the transference number can be used to compute the ionic equivalent conductances ℓ_c^o

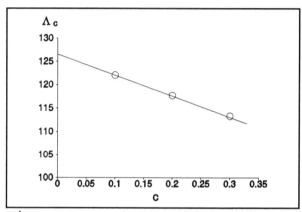

Figure P6-1 for Problem 6.3

and ℓ_a^o since $t_{a^-} = \dfrac{\ell_a^o}{\Lambda_o}$ and $t_{c^+} = \dfrac{\ell_c^o}{\Lambda_o}$ are

the fraction of current carried by the anion and cation respectively.

$t_{c+}^o = 0.396 = \dfrac{\ell_c^o}{126.45}$; $\ell_c^o = 50.07$ mho cm^2/Eq

Therefore, since $\Lambda_o = \ell_a^o + \ell_c^o$; $\ell_a^o = 126.45 - 50.07 = 76.38$ mho cm^2/Eq; $t_{a-}^o = 1 - 0.396 = 0.604$

PROBLEM 6.4. (a) The data are plotted in Figure P6 − 2.
By extrapolation, Λ_c for 1 M NaCl is 83 mho cm^2/Eq;
By least squares, $\Lambda_c = 83.54 - 23.1c$; $r^2 = 1.000$

Table P6-1 for Problem 6.3

$\sqrt{c}$	0.3	0.2	0.1
Λ_c	113.34	117.70	122.08

Therefore, the intercept at which c = 0 is 83.54 ohm^{-1} cm^2/Eq = Λ_c for 1 M NaCl.

(b) From the equation obtained in problem 6.3,

Λ_c(1 molar) = 126.45 − 43.70 $\sqrt{1}$

= 82.75 ohm^{-1} cm^2/Eq. This result checks with the value obtained above, viz, 83.54 ohm^{-1} cm^2/Eq.

(c) Chloral hydrate interacts with the anion Cl$^-$ of NaCl to form a hydrogen bonded complex,

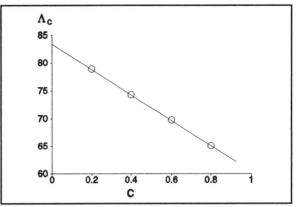

Figure P6–2 for Problem 6.4

$$Cl_3C - CH \overset{\displaystyle OH \cdots}{\underset{\displaystyle OH \cdots}{\Big\langle}} Cl^-$$

and the concentration of free Cl$^-$ decreases. The size of the anionic complex in aqueous solution being much larger than the free chloride ion, the velocity of the complexed ion decreases and the fraction of the total current carried by the anion is lowered. This most likely results in a decrease in the equivalent conductance of the solution as the concentration of chloral hydrate increases.

The interaction of chloral hydrate with halide ions to form hydrogen bonded complexes, as demonstrated here, may be of importance in the anesthetic (hypnotic and sedative) action of these systems; and the hydrogen bridging of chloral hydrate with various proton acceptors is under continued investigation[a].

PROBLEM 6.5. π = mRT = 1 x 0.0821 x 273.15 = 22.4 atm.

$$i = \frac{real}{ideal} = \frac{24.8}{22.4} = 1.11$$

PROBLEM 6.6. We must decrease the freezing point of ice from 0°C to − 12.22°C (10°F); ΔT_f = 12.22°

The van't Hoff factor i for CaCl$_2$ is given by equation (6−34), i = 1 + a(v − 1).

CaCl$_2$ dissociates into 3 ions, therefore

---

[a]   P. Hobza, F. Mulder and C. Sandorfy, J. Am. Chem. Soc. 104, 925, 1982. M. Otagiri et. al. Chem. Pharm. Bull. 23, 3228, 1975. E. M. Schulman et al, J. Am. Chem. Soc. 98, 3793, 1976. C. Brisson et al., J. Mol. Struct. 68, 137, 1980

$$i = 1 + 0.8(3 - 1) = 2.6$$

To reduce the temperature of frozen water (ice) at $0°C$ to $-12.22°C$ requires a molal concentration, m of $CaCl_2$:

$$m = \frac{\Delta T_f}{i\,K_f} = \frac{12.22}{2.6 \times 1.86} = 2.53 \text{ mole } CaCl_2/kg \text{ water}$$

2.53 mole/kg x 110.99 g/mole = 280.8 g $CaCl_2$/kg water

The volume of the sidewalk is:

$$50 \times 4 = 200 \text{ ft} \times 0.5 \text{ inches} \times \frac{1\ ft}{12\ inches} = 8.33 \text{ ft}^3$$

From a handbook, 8.33 ft^3 x 28.317 liters/ft^3 = 235.88 liters of ice;

235.88 x 10^3 ml x 0.9973 g/ml = 235243 g of ice or 235.2 kg of ice

We need (280.8 g $CaCl_2$ /kg ice) x 235.2 kg ice = 66044 g or 66 kg of $CaCl_2$ or 66 kg x 2.2 lb/kg = 145 lb

PROBLEM 6.7. (a) NaCl added to water raises its boiling point. The boiling point of water will occur at a higher temperature and should cook the food to a softer consistency (as compared to unsalted boiling water).

 (b) In order to get a significant rise in the boiling point, say 5°, the amount of NaCl needed is (taking i ≅ 2 for NaCl)

$$m = \frac{\Delta T_b}{i\,K_b} = \frac{5}{2 \times 0.51} = 4.9 \text{ m}$$

4.9 moles/kg H_2O x 58.44 g/mole NaCl = 286.356 g/kg ≈ 286 g/liter of NaCl.

However, this concentration is too salty. Even to get a rise of 1°, the concentration needed of NaCl would be too salty.

PROBLEM 6.8. (a) Aureomycin:

$$1\% \text{ solution} = \frac{10\ g/\ell}{544\ g/mole} = 0.0184 \text{ mole/liter} \approx 0.0184 \text{ mole/kg } H_2O$$

$$i = \frac{\Delta T_f}{m\,K_f} = \frac{0.06}{0.0184 \times 1.86} = 1.753$$

From equation (6–35): $\alpha = \dfrac{i - 1}{v - 1} = \dfrac{1.753 - 1}{2 - 1} = 0.753$

Therefore, aureomycin hydrochloride is 75 per cent dissociated

(b) (atropine$^+$)$_2$SO$_4^=$ ⇌ 2 atropine$^+$ + SO$_4^=$; $v = 3$

$$m \approx \frac{10}{694.82} = 0.0144 \text{ m}; \qquad i = \frac{0.07}{0.0144 \times 1.86} = 2.614$$

$$\alpha = \frac{2.614 - 1}{3 - 1} = \frac{1.614}{2} = 0.807 \text{ or } 81\%$$

(c) For physostigmine,

$$(\text{physostigmine}^+)(\text{salicylate}^-) \rightleftarrows \text{physostigmine}^+ + \text{salicylate}^-$$

$$\nu = 2; \quad m = \frac{10}{413.46} = 0.0242; \quad i = \frac{0.09}{0.0242 \times 1.86} = 1.999$$

$$\alpha = \frac{1.999 - 1}{2 - 1} = 0.999 \text{ or } 99.9\%$$

(d) Aureomycin hydrochloride is 75 % dissociated, atropine sulfate is 81% dissociated, and physostigmine salicylate is 99.9 % dissociated.

PROBLEM 6.9. $\alpha = \dfrac{\Lambda_c}{\Lambda_o} = \dfrac{113.24 \ ohm^{-1} \ cm^2}{126.45 \ ohm^{-1} \ cm^2} = 0.896$

$i = 1 + \alpha(\nu - 1) = 1 + 0.896 (2 - 1) = 1.896$

$\Delta T_f = iK_f m = 1.896 \times 1.86 \times 0.09 = 0.32$ degrees.

PROBLEM 6.10. $\alpha = \dfrac{\Lambda_c}{\Lambda_o} = \dfrac{1.104}{400} = 0.00276$ or 0.28%

PROBLEM 6.11. (a) The vapor pressure of pure water at 100°C is 760 mm Hg (equal to the atmospheric pressure)

Activity of water $= \dfrac{p_1}{p_1^o} = \dfrac{721}{760} = 0.949$

(b) Activity of methanol $= \dfrac{703}{760} = 0.925$

(c) Activity of chlorine $= \dfrac{9.30}{10} = 0.930$

(d) Activity of formic acid $= \dfrac{32.2}{40} = 0.805$

PROBLEM 6.12. (a) The molality of $CaCl_2$ is

$$\frac{250 \ g/kg \ H_2O}{110.99 \ g/mole} = 2.25 \text{ mole/(kg water)}$$

ν is roughly 3 and $\Delta p_1 = 0.018 \ i \ p^o \ m = 0.018 \times 3 \times 23.8 \times 2.25 = 2.89$ mm Hg;

$23.8 - 2.89 = 20.91$ torr

(b) $\quad a_1 = \dfrac{p_1}{p^o} = \dfrac{20.91}{23.8} = 0.879$

Mole fraction of water:

$1 \text{ kg H}_2\text{O} = \dfrac{1000 \ g}{18.015 \ g/mole} = 55.51 \text{ mole} ; \quad X_1 = \dfrac{55.51}{2.25 + 55.51} = 0.961$

$\gamma_1 = \dfrac{a_1}{X_1} = \dfrac{0.879}{0.961} = 0.915$

PROBLEM 6.13. **(a)** 15 g in 100 g water = 150 g/kg water

$\text{molality} = \dfrac{150 \ g/kg}{40.01 \ g/mole} = 3.75 \text{ mole/(kg water)}$

$\Delta p = 0.018 \ i \ p^o \ m = 0.018 \times 2 \times 23.8 \times 3.75 = 3.21 \text{ mm Hg}$

The vapor pressure of the solution is $23.8 - 3.21 = 20.59$ mm Hg (torr)

(b) $\quad a_1 = \dfrac{p_1}{p_1^o} = \dfrac{20.59}{23.8} = 0.865$

$\text{Moles of water} = \dfrac{100 - 15}{18.015} = 4.718; \quad \text{moles of NaOH} = \dfrac{15}{40.01} = 0.375$

$\text{Mole fraction of water} = \dfrac{4.718}{4.718 + 0.375} = 0.926$

$\gamma_1 = \dfrac{a_1}{X_1} = \dfrac{0.865}{0.926} = 0.934$

PROBLEM 6.14. The molality of the glucose solution is $\dfrac{100 \ g/kg}{180.16} = 0.555$ mole/kg

$\Delta p = 0.018 \times 23.8 \times 0.555 = 0.2378 \text{ torr}$

$p_1 = p_1^o - \Delta p = 23.8 - 0.2378 = 23.562 \text{ torr}$

The mole fraction of glucose is $X_2 = \dfrac{0.555}{0.555 + 55.5} = 0.0099$

The mole fraction of water is $X_1 = 1 - 0.0099 = 0.990$

$\gamma_1 = \dfrac{p_1}{X_1 \ p_1^o} = \dfrac{23.562}{0.990 \times 23.8} = 1.000$

$a_1 = \gamma_1 X_1 = 1.000 \times 0.990 = 0.990$

Thus in a 10 g/100 ml H_2O solution of glucose, the activity and activity coefficients may both be taken as approximately 1.000

PROBLEM 6.15. $\mu = 0.01 + 0.01 = 0.02$ since both are 1:1 electrolytes

$$\log \gamma_{\pm} = -Az_{+}z_{-} \sqrt{\mu} = -0.51 \times 1 \times 1 \sqrt{0.02} = -0.07212 \; ; \quad \gamma_{\pm} = 0.85$$

PROBLEM 6.16. Both are 1:1 electrolytes, and the ionic strength is $\mu = 0.05 + 0.05 = 0.1$. The concentration is larger than 0.02 M, so we use the extension of the Debye−Hückel equation:

$$\log \gamma_{\pm} = -\frac{A z_{+}z_{-} \sqrt{\mu}}{1 + \sqrt{\mu}} = \frac{-0.51 \times 1 \times 1 \sqrt{0.1}}{1 + \sqrt{0.1}} = -0.1225 \; ; \quad \gamma_{\pm} = 0.75$$

PROBLEM 6.17. (a) First, we calculate the ionic strength of the 0.02 M solution of neomycin sulfate, $(\text{neomycin}^{+})_2 SO_4^{=}$
The concentration of $2(\text{neomycin})^{+}$ is 0.02×2 , and the concentration of $SO_4^{=}$ is 0.02.

The ionic strength is $\mu = \frac{1}{2}[(0.02 \times 2 \times 1^2) + (0.02 \times 2^2)] = 0.06$

To get a total ionic strength of 0.09,

$\mu_{total} = \mu_{neomycin\ SO_4^{=}} + \mu_{CaCl_2} \; ; \quad \mu_{CaCl_2} = 0.09 - 0.06 = 0.03$

The concentration, c, of $CaCl_2$ needed to get an ionic strength of 0.03 is obtained from the equation:

$$\mu_{CaCl_2} = 0.03 = \frac{1}{2}[(2 \times c \times 1^2) + (c \times 2^2)] = \frac{1}{2}(2c + 4c) = 3c$$

where the unknown concentration of Cl^{-} is $2 \times c$ and the unknown concentration of Ca^{++} is c; solving for c, we get c = 0.01. We need a 0.01 M solution of $CaCl_2$ to produce a total ionic strength of 0.09.

(b) $\log \gamma_{\pm} = -Az_{+}z_{-} \sqrt{\mu} = -0.51 \times 2 \times 1 \sqrt{0.09} = -0.306 \; ; \quad \gamma_{\pm} = 0.494$

$$a_{\pm} = \gamma_{\pm}(c_{+}^{m} c_{-}^{n})^{1/(m + n)} = 0.494[(0.02 \times 2)^2 (0.02)]^{1/3} = 0.0157$$

Using the extension of the Debye−Hückel equation:

$$\log \gamma_{\pm} = -\frac{0.51 \times 2 \sqrt{0.09}}{1 + \sqrt{0.09}} = -0.235; \quad \gamma_{\pm} = 0.582$$

In this case, $a_{\pm} = 0.582[(0.02 \times 2)^2 (0.02)]^{1/3} = 0.0185$
The results from the two equations are different. The solution has an ionic strength above 0.02, so the value of the denominator is not unity. In addition, $\sqrt{\mu}$ in the numerator has to be multiplied by 2 because it is a unibivalent electrolyte. For this concentration, we should use the extension of the Debye−Hückel equation.

PROBLEM 6.18. (a) The ionic strength is

$$\mu = \frac{1}{2}[(0.274 \times 1^2) + (0.274 \times 1^2)] = 0.274$$

We use equation (6 – 60) because μ is larger than 0.1.

$$\log \gamma_\pm = \frac{-0.51\sqrt{0.274}}{1 + \sqrt{0.274}} = -0.1753 \; ; \quad \gamma_\pm = 0.668$$

$$a_\pm = \gamma_\pm (c_+ \cdot c_-)^{1/2} = 0.668 \,(0.274 \times 0.274)^{1/2} = 0.183$$

(b) The ionic strength of brequinar in the solution is now 0.245 (the same value as the concentration); μ for NaCl is also the same as concentration, 0.01.
The total ionic strength is

$$\mu = 0.01 + 0.245 = 0.255$$

$$\log \gamma_\pm = \frac{-0.51 \times \sqrt{0.255}}{1 + \sqrt{0.255}} = -0.17112 \; ; \quad \gamma_\pm = 0.674$$

$$a_\pm = \gamma_\pm(c_+ \cdot c_-)^{1/2} = 0.674 (0.245 \times 0.245)^{1/2} = 0.165$$

PROBLEM 6.19. For sodium phenobarbital, a 1:1 electrolyte:

$$\mu = \frac{1}{2}[(0.003 \times 1^2) + (0.003 \times 1^2)] = 0.003$$

For sodium acetate,

$$\mu = \frac{1}{2}[(0.2 \times 1^2) + (0.2 \times 1^2)] = 0.2$$

For acetic acid, the concentration of dissociated species is
$0.30 \times 0.008 = 0.0024$, and the ionic strength is

$$\mu = \frac{1}{2}[(0.0024 \times 1^2) + (0.0024 \times 1^2)] = 0.0024$$

The total ionic strength is $\mu = 0.003 + 0.2 + 0.0024 = 0.205$

PROBLEM 6.20. For 0.05 M $AlCl_3$, $[Al^{3+}] = 0.05$; $[Cl^-] = 0.05 \times 3 = 0.15$
For 0.2 M Na_2HPO_4, $[Na^+] = 0.2 \times 2 = 0.4$; $[HPO_4^=] = 0.2$

$$\mu = \frac{1}{2}[(0.05)(3)^2 + (0.15)(1)^2 + (0.4)(1)^2 + (0.2)(2)^2] = 0.90$$

PROBLEM 6.21. (See Table P6 – 2)

$$\frac{8.6g}{58.45g/mole} = 0.14713 \text{ mole NaCl}; \quad \frac{0.3}{74.55} = 0.00402 \text{ mole KCl}$$

$$\frac{0.33}{147.03} = 0.00224 \text{ mole } CaCl_2 \; ;$$

Table P6 − 2 for Problem 6.21.

Ringer's Solution		
	grams	molecular weight
NaCl	8.6	58.45
KCl	0.3	74.55
$CaCl_2 \cdot 2H_2O$	0.33	147.03
H_2O qs ad	1000	

$$\mu = \frac{1}{2}[(0.14713)(1)^2 + (0.14713)(1)^2 + (0.00402)(1)^2 + (0.00402)(1)^2 + (0.00224)(2)^2$$

$$+ (0.00224 \times 2)(1)^2] = 0.16$$

PROBLEM 6.22. (a)   The molality of the solution is

$$m = \frac{40\ g}{297.85\ g/mole} = 0.13430\ ;\quad i = \frac{0.423}{1.86 \times 0.13430} = 1.69$$

(b) $g = \dfrac{i}{\nu} = \dfrac{1.69}{2} = 0.85$

(c) $L = g\ \nu \times 1.86 = 0.85 \times 2 \times 1.86 = 3.16$

PROBLEM 6.23. (a) $\alpha = \dfrac{\Lambda_c}{\Lambda_o} = \dfrac{48.15}{390.7} = 0.12$

(b) $i = 1 + \alpha(2 - 1) = 1 + 0.12(2 - 1) = 1.12$

(c) $L = i\ K_f = 1.12 \times 1.86 = 2.1$

PROBLEM 6.24. $i = \dfrac{L}{K_f} = \dfrac{1.90}{1.86} = 1.02$

$$m = \frac{\pi}{iRT} = \frac{\left(\dfrac{1182}{760}\right) atm}{1.02 \times 0.0821 \times 310} = 0.06$$

$$\Delta T_f = 1.9 \times 0.06 = 0.11°\ ;\quad \alpha = \frac{i - 1}{\nu - 1} = \frac{1.02 - 1}{2 - 1} = 0.02$$

The degree of ionization is 0.02 or 2%

PROBLEM 6.25. The millimolality of sodium iodide is 0.25 molar x 1000 = 250 millimoles/kg;

Milliosmolality = i x millimolality = 1.86 x 250 = 465 mOsm/kg

ΔT_f = K_f x osmolality = 1.86 x 0.465 Osm/kg = 0.86°

$NaHCO_3$ is also a 1:1 electrolyte;

1.86 x 250 millimolal = 465 mOsm/kg ; ΔT_f = 1.86 x 0.465 Osm/kg = 0.86°

$CaCl_2$ is a 2:1 electrolyte, i = 2.6

2.6 x 250 = 650 mOsm/kg ; ΔT_f = 2.6 x 0.650 Osm/kg = 1.69°

Griseofulvin and pentobarbital are nonelectrolytes, i = 1. The osmolality for both compounds is: 1 x 340 millimoles = 340 mOsm/kg

Their freezing point depression is: ΔT_f = 1.86 x 0.340 Osm/kg = 0.63°

For the pentobarbital solution, i = 1. The osmotic pressure of an osmolal solution is 24.4 atm.

π = 0.340 Osm/kg x 24.4 = 8.3 atm.

The osmotic pressure of the $NaHCO_3$ solution is

π = 0.465 Osm/kg x 24.4 = 11.3 atm

PROBLEM 6.26. Using equation (6 – 66):

mOsm/liter = mOsm/kg[ρ_1^o(1 – 0.001 $\overline{v_2^o}$)]

where ρ_1^o is the density of water, 0.997 at 25°C and $\overline{v_2^o}$ is the partial molar volume of KBr = 33.97,

mOsm/liter = 223 mOsm/kg[0.997 g/cm³(1 – 0.001 x 33.97)] = 214.8 mOsm/liter.

PROBLEM 6.27. (a) The activity is computed from the vapor pressure of the pure solvent and the vapor pressure of the solution, i.e. $a_1 = \dfrac{p_1}{p_1^o}$; the activity coefficient is

$\gamma_1 = \dfrac{a_1}{X_1}$. For example, when X_1 = 1, $a_1 = \dfrac{344.5}{344.5}$ = 1 and γ_1 = 1. For X_1 = 0.950,

$a_1 = \dfrac{327.0}{344.5}$ = 0.949 and $\gamma_1 = \dfrac{0.949}{0.950}$ = 0.999. The results are shown in Table P6 – 3

Table P6 – 3 for Problem 6.27.

X_1	1.000	0.950	0.925	0.878	0.710	0.575
a_1	1.000	0.949	0.920	0.870	0.670	0.504
γ_1	1.000	0.999	0.995	0.991	0.943	0.877

(b) The partial pressure, p_1, is plotted against the mole fraction, X_1, in Figure P6 – 3.
The escaping tendency of acetone is reduced below the Raoult law value in these mixtures. Figure P6 – 3 and Table P6 – 3 show negative deviation from Raoult's law over most of the curve; therefore the intermolecular interaction between chloroform and acetone is greater than that in an ideal solution.

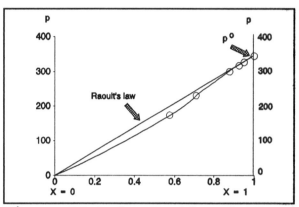

Figure P6-3 for Problem 6.27

PROBLEM 6.28. The calculations are as in problem 6.27. The results are presented in Table P6 – 4.

Table P6 – 4 for Problem 6.28.

X_1	1.000	0.942	0.740	0.497
a_1	1.000	0.938	0.689	0.433
γ_1	1.000	0.996	0.931	0.871

CHAPTER 7
Ionic Equilibria

PROBLEM 7.1.(a) $[H_3O^+]$ = antilog($-$pH) = 2.88×10^{-3} M

(b) $[H_3O^+] = \dfrac{C_a + \sqrt{C_a^2 + 4K_w}}{2} = \dfrac{7.93 \times 10^{-4} + \sqrt{(7.93 \times 10^{-4})^2 + 4 \times 10^{-14}}}{2}$

$= 7.93 \times 10^{-4}$ M , so $[H_3O^+] = C_a$; pH = 3.10

(c) $[H_3O^+]$ = antilog(-8.75) = 1.78×10^{-9} M

$[OH^-] = \dfrac{1.0 \times 10^{-14}}{1.78 \times 10^{-9}} = 5.62 \times 10^{-6}$

(d) $[H_3O^+] = \dfrac{C_a + \sqrt{C_a^2 + 4K_w}}{2} = \dfrac{0.00379 + \sqrt{(0.00379)^2 + 4 \times 10^{-14}}}{2}$

$= 3.79 \times 10^{-3}$ M ; $[H_3O^+] = C_a$; pH = 2.42; pOH = 14 $-$ 2.42 = 11.58

(e) pOH = $-$log $[OH^-]$ = $-$log (0.00915) = 2.04; pH = 14 $-$ 2.04 = 11.96

(f) $H_2SO_4 \rightarrow SO_4^{2-} + 2H^+$

$[H_3O^+]$ = 2 x 2.37×10^{-3} = 4.74×10^{-3} M ; pH = $-$log(4.74×10^{-3}) = 2.32

(g) 0.017 M of HCl will neutralize 0.017 M NaOH to yield 0.017 M NaCl. The pH of water (pH = 7) will be affected by the ionic strength of NaCl. Since the concentration is <0.02 M, the mean ionic activity coefficient is

$\log \gamma_{\pm} = -Az_+z_- \sqrt{\mu} = -0.51 \times 1 \times 1 \sqrt{0.017} = -0.0665$; $\gamma_{\pm} = 0.858$

pH = $-$log($\gamma_{\pm}$C) = $-$log(0.858 x 1 x 10^{-7}) = 7.07

(h) $\log \gamma_{\pm} = \dfrac{-Az_+z_-\sqrt{\mu}}{1 + \sqrt{\mu}} = \dfrac{-0.51 \times 1 \times 1\sqrt{0.034}}{1 + \sqrt{0.034}} -0.0794$; $\gamma_{\pm} = 0.833$

pH = $-$log($\gamma_{\pm}$C) = $-$log(0.833 x 1 x 10^{-7}) = 7.08, where $[H^+]$ is 1 x 10^{-7}

(i) 0.14% w/v is 1.4 g/(232.23 g/mole) = 6.03×10^{-3} M

$[H_3O^+] = \sqrt{K_a C_a} = \sqrt{(3.9 \times 10^{-8})(0.00603)} = 1.53 \times 10^{-5}$; pH = 4.81

(j) They will react to yield sodium acetate, a salt of a weak acid and a strong base. CH_3COONa dissociates into Na^+ and CH_3COO^-:

$CH_3COO^- + H_2O \rightleftharpoons CH_3-COOH + [OH^-]$

$[OH^-] = \sqrt{K_b C_b} = \sqrt{(5.71 \times 10^{-10})(0.02)} = 3.38 \times 10^{-6}$ M where $K_b = \dfrac{1.0 \times 10^{-14}}{1.75 \times 10^{-5}} = 5.71 \times 10^{-10}$ M (K_a for acetic acid is 1.75×10^{-5} M from

Table 7 – 1)

$pOH = -\log(3.38 \times 10^{-6}) = 5.47$; $pH = pK_w - pOH = 14 - 5.47 = 8.53$

$[H_3O^+] = \text{antilog}(-8.53) = 2.95 \times 10^{-9}$ M

(k) $pH = 14 - 6.82 = 7.18$; $[OH^-] = \text{antilog}(-6.82) = 1.51 \times 10^{-7}$

(l) In this dilute solution, equation (7 – 85) must be used intead of equation (7 – 86).

$$[H_3O^+] = \frac{C_a + \sqrt{C_a^2 + 4K_w}}{2}$$

$$[H_3O^+] = \frac{5.0 \times 10^{-8} + \sqrt{(5.0 \times 10^{-8})^2 + (4 \times 10^{-14})}}{2} = 1.28 \times 10^{-7}\ \text{M}$$

$$pH = -\log(1.28 \times 10^{-7}) = 6.89\ ;\quad pOH = 7.11$$

(m) $[H_3O^+] = \sqrt{K_a C_a} = \sqrt{(1.77 \times 10^{-4})(0.06)} = 3.26 \times 10^{-3}$ M ; $pH = 2.49$

PROBLEM 7.2. Sulfathiazole reacts with NaOH to give sodium sulfathiazole. The volume (ml) of acid (free sulfathiazole) neutralized by NaOH is:

$VM = V'M'$; $0.005 \times V = 57 \times 0.003$; $V = 34.2$ ml of the 100 ml are now sodium sulfathiazole. The volume of free acid is $100 - 34.2 = 65.8$ ml.

Therefore, after the addition of 57 ml of 0.003 M NaOH, we have 34.2 ml of 0.005 M sodium sulfathiazole and 65.8 ml of 0.005 M sulfathiazole solution. We use the Henderson – Hasselbalch equation (equation(8-8)) to calculate the pH of the solution. Since both salt and acid are 0.005 M, the ratio of the two is 34.2/65.8:

$$pH = pK_a + \log\frac{[salt]}{[acid]} = 7.12 + \log\frac{34.2}{65.8} = 6.84$$

where 7.12 is the pK_a of sulfathiazole (acid) ; $pOH = 14 - 6.84 = 7.16$

PROBLEM 7.3. (a) Using equation (13 – 95),

Fraction of free phenobarbital, a weak acid:

$$\frac{1}{1 + 10^{(pH - pK_a)}} = \frac{1}{1 + 10^{(8 - 7.48)}} = 0.23 \text{ or } 23\ \% \text{ nonionized}$$

(b) Fraction of free cocaine, a weak base:

$$\frac{1}{1 + 10^{(pK_a - pH)}} = \frac{1}{1 + 10^{(8.41 - 8)}} = 0.28 \text{ or } 28\ \% \text{ nonionized}$$

PROBLEM 7.4. $C_a = 5.0 \ g/95.12 \ (g/mole) = 0.0526 \ mole/100 \ ml = 0.526 \ M$

$[H_3O^+] = \sqrt{K_a C_a} = \sqrt{(1.0 \times 10^{-10})(0.526)} = 7.25 \times 10^{-6} \ M \ ; \ pH = 5.14$

$[OH^-] = \dfrac{K_w}{[H_3O^+]} = \dfrac{1.0 \times 10^{-14} \ M^2}{7.25 \times 10^{-6} \ M} = 1.38 \times 10^{-9} \ M$

PROBLEM 7.5. The approximate equation gives:

$[H_3O^+] = \sqrt{K_a C_a} = \sqrt{(1.75 \times 10^{-5})(0.001)} = 1.32 \times 10^{-4} \ M \ ; \ pH = 3.88$

The more exact equation (7–98) gives:

$$[H_3O^+] = \dfrac{-1.75 \times 10^{-5} + \sqrt{(1.75 \times 10^{-5})^2 + 4(1.75 \times 10^{-5})(0.001)}}{2} =$$

$= 1.24 \times 10^{-4} \ M \ ; \qquad pH = 3.91$

PROBLEM 7.6. The concentration of weak acid, BH^+ (morphine cation) is two times the concentration of salt added (see Example 7–13):

$$(BH^+)_2 SO_4^{2-} \rightleftharpoons 2 \ BH^+ + SO_4^{2-}$$

$C_a = 2 \times C_{salt} = \dfrac{2 \times 10 \ g/\ell}{668.76 \ g/mole} = 2.99 \times 10^{-2} \ M$

$K_a = \dfrac{1 \times 10^{-14}}{7.4 \times 10^{-7}} = 1.35 \times 10^{-8} \ ; \ [H_3O^+] = \sqrt{K_a C_s}$

$= \sqrt{(1.35 \times 10^{-8})(2.99 \times 10^{-2})} = 2.01 \times 10^{-5}; \ pH = 4.70$

PROBLEM 7.7. A solution 1:200 corresponds to 5 g/liter. The molecular weight of ephedrine is 165.23, and the molar concentration is (5 g/liter)/(165.23 g/mole) = 0.03 M

$[OH^-] = \sqrt{K_b C_b} = \sqrt{(2.3 \times 10^{-5})(0.03)} = 8.31 \times 10^{-4} \ M$

$[H_3O^+] = \dfrac{1.0 \times 10^{-14}}{8.31 \times 10^{-4}} = 1.20 \times 10^{-11} \ ; \ pH = 10.92$

PROBLEM 7.8. Tartaric acid has two dissociation constants. Since $K_1 \gg K_2$ (see Example 7–18), using equation (7–99).

$[H_3O^+] = \sqrt{K_a C_a} = \sqrt{(9.6 \times 10^{-4})(0.01)} = 3.1 \times 10^{-3} \ M$

Since C_a is not much greater than $[H_3O^+]$, we use the quadratic equation (7–112):

$$[H_3O^+] = \frac{-K_a + \sqrt{K_a^2 + 4 K_a C_a}}{2} =$$

$$\frac{-9.6 \times 10^{-4} + \sqrt{(9.6 \times 10^{-4})^2 + 4(9.6 \times 10^{-4})(0.01)}}{2} = 2.66 \times 10^{-3} \text{ M}$$

pH = 2.58

PROBLEM 7.9. Using equation (7 – 105):

$$[OH^-] = \sqrt{K_b C_b} = \sqrt{(7.6 \times 10^{-7})(0.01)} = 8.72 \times 10^{-5} \, M$$

Since $C_b \gg [OH^-]$, the assumptions hold; pOH = 4.06 and

pH = 14 – pOH = 14 – 4.06 = 9.94

PROBLEM 7.10. The concentration of acetic acid is C_1 and for formic acid is C_2. Using equation (7 – 124):

$$[H_3O^+] = \sqrt{K_1 C_1 + K_2 C_2} = \sqrt{(1.75 \times 10^{-5})(0.1) + (1.77 \times 10^{-4})(0.1)}$$
$$= 4.41 \times 10^{-3} \text{ M}; \; \text{pH} = 2.36$$

PROBLEM 7.11. Using equation (7 – 124) where $K_1 = 3.3 \times 10^{-7}$ and $K_2 = 1 \times 10^{-5}$:

$$[H_3O^+] = \sqrt{K_1 C_1 + K_2 C_2} = \sqrt{(3.3 \times 10^{-7})(0.01) + (1 \times 10^{-5})(0.05)}$$
$$= 7.094 \times 10^{-4}; \; \text{pH} = -\log(7.094 \times 10^{-4}) = 3.15$$

PROBLEM 7.12. (a) $[H_3O^+] = [OH^-] + [NH_3]$

(b) $[H_3O^+] + 2[H_3PO_4] + [H_2PO_4^-] = [OH^-] + [NH_3] + [PO_4^{3-}]$

PROBLEM 7.13. $K_1 = 10^{-2.3} = 5.01 \times 10^{-3}$; $K_2 = 10^{-4.9} = 1.26 \times 10^{-5}$;

$$[H_3O^+] = \sqrt{K_1 K_2} = \sqrt{(5.01 \times 10^{-3})(1.26 \times 10^{-5})} = 2.51 \times 10^{-4} \, M; \quad pH = 3.6$$

PROBLEM 7.14. $K_1 = 10^{-2.1} = 7.94 \times 10^{-3}$; $K_2 = 10^{-6.5} = 3.16 \times 10^{-7}$

$$[H_3O^+] = \sqrt{K_1 K_2} = \sqrt{(7.94 \times 10^{-3})(3.16 \times 10^{-7})} = 5.01 \times 10^{-5} \, M; \quad pH = 4.3$$

PROBLEM 7.15. Using the more exact equation (7 – 114):

$$[H_3O^+] = \sqrt{\frac{K_1 K_2 C_{ab}}{K_1 + C_{ab}}} \quad \sqrt{\frac{(6.92 \times 10^{-4})(1.17 \times 10^{-7})(4.7 \times 10^{-3})}{6.92 \times 10^{-4} + 4.7 \times 10^{-3}}} =$$

8.40×10^{-6} M; pH = 5.08

Using the approximate equation (7 – 115),

$$[H_3O^+] = \sqrt{K_1 K_2} = \sqrt{(6.92 \times 10^{-4})(1.17 \times 10^{-7})} = 8.998 \times 10^{-6} \text{ M}$$

$$pH = -\log[H_3O^+] = -\log(8.998 \times 10^{-6}) = 5.05$$

PROBLEM 7.16.

$$[H_3O^+] = \frac{K_a C_a}{C_b} = \frac{(1.75 \times 10^{-5})(0.1)}{0.02} = 8.75 \times 10^{-5}; \text{ pH} = 4.06$$

PROBLEM 7.17. (a)

$$K_1 = K_{a(NH_4^+)} = \frac{K_w}{K_{b(NH_4^+)}} = \frac{1.0 \times 10^{-14}}{1.74 \times 10^{-5}} = 5.75 \times 10^{-10}$$

$$K_2 = K_{a(\text{boric acid})} = 5.8 \times 10^{-10}$$

$$[H_3O^+] = \sqrt{K_1 K_2} = \sqrt{(5.75 \times 10^{-10})(5.8 \times 10^{-10})} = 5.77 \times 10^{-10}; \text{ pH} = 9.24$$

(b) $K_1 = K_{a(NH_4^+)} = 5.75 \times 10^{-10}$; $K_2 = K_a$ (propionic acid) $= 1.34 \times 10^{-5}$

$$[H_3O^+] = \sqrt{(5.75 \times 10^{-10})(1.34 \times 10^{-5})} = 8.78 \times 10^{-8} \text{ M; } pH = 7.06$$

PROBLEM 7.18.

$$(NH_4^+)_3 PO_4 \rightarrow 3\,NH_4^+ + PO_4^{3-}$$
$$NH_4^+ + PO_4^{3-} \rightleftharpoons HPO_2^{2-} + NH_3$$
$$\quad A_1 \qquad B_2 \qquad A_2 \qquad B_1$$

$$[H_3O^+] = \sqrt{n K_1 K_2} = \sqrt{3(5.75 \times 10^{-10})(2.1 \times 10^{-13})} = 1.90 \times 10^{-11} ; \text{ pH} = 10.72$$

where K_1 is the K_a of NH_4^+ and K_2 is the third ionization constant of phosphoric acid.

PROBLEM 7.19. Na_3 citrate $\rightarrow 3\,Na^+ +$ citrate^{3-}

$$H_2 \text{ succ } + \text{ citrate}^{3-} \rightarrow H \text{ succ}^- + H \text{ citrate}^{2-}$$

$$H \text{ succ}^- + H \text{ citrate}^{2-} \rightleftharpoons \text{ succ}^{2-} + H_2 \text{ citrate}^-$$

Acid 1   Acid 2

$K_1 = 2.3 \times 10^{-6}$ $K_2 = 1.7 \times 10^{-5}$

$$[H_3O^+] = \sqrt{K_1 K_2} = \sqrt{(2.3 \times 10^{-6})(1.7 \times 10^{-5})} = 6.25 \times 10^{-6}; \text{ pH} = 5.20$$

where K_1 is the second ionization constant of succinic acid and K_2 is the second ionization constant of sodium citrate.

PROBLEM 7.20. (a) $K_b = \dfrac{[BH^+]\,[OH^-]}{[B]} = 1 \times 10^{-5}$

Let x be the amount of ionized, $[BH^+]$ and $[OH^-]$ species in solution so that un-ionized [B] is

$(0.003 - x);\quad \dfrac{x \cdot x}{0.003 - x} = \dfrac{x^2}{0.003 - x} = 1 \times 10^{-5}$

Rearranging terms, $x^2 + (1 \cdot 10^{-5})x - (3 \cdot 10^{-8}) = 0$,

$x = \dfrac{-1\times10^{-5} \pm \sqrt{(1\times10^{-5})^2 + (4\times3\times10^{-8})}}{2} = \begin{pmatrix} 1.68\times10^{-4} \\ -1.78\times10^{-4} \end{pmatrix}$

We take the positive root, $x = 1.68 \times 10^{-4}$. At equilibrium we have 1.68×10^{-4} moles of $[BH^+]$ and 1.68×10^{-4} moles of OH^-.

The concentration of ionized aminophylline is 1.68×10^{-4} mole/liter.

The concentration of un-ionized aminophylline is:

$[0.003 - (1.68 \times 10^{-4})] = 2.83 \times 10^{-3}$ mole/liter

(b) $[OH^-] = 1.68 \times 10^{-4}$; pOH = 3.77

pH = pK_w − pOH = 14 − 3.77 = 10.23

PROBLEM 7.21.

$[H_3O^+] = \sqrt{\dfrac{K_a K_w}{C_b}} = \sqrt{\dfrac{(3.3\times10^{-7})(1.0\times10^{-14})}{0.5}} = 8.12 \times 10^{-11}$ M; pH = 10.09

PROBLEM 7.22. (a)   Using equation (13-77):

% ionized acid = $\dfrac{100}{1 + antilog(pK_a - pH)}$

$= \dfrac{100}{1 + antilog\ (3.49 - 3.20)} = 33.9\ \%$

(b) $\Delta G^\circ = 2.303\ RT\ pK = 2.303 \times 1.9872 \times 298.15 \times 3.49 = 4762$ cal/mole

(c) $\Delta G = \Delta G^\circ + 2.303\ RT\ \log Q$

$AH \rightleftarrows A^- + H^+$;   33.9% of 0.00167 M = $5.66 \times 10^{-4} = [A^-]$

$Q = \dfrac{[A^-]\,[H^+]}{[AH]} = \dfrac{(5.66\times10^{-4})(5.66\times10^{-4})}{(0.00167) - (5.66\times10^{-4})} = 2.9\times10^{-4}$

$\Delta G = 4762 + [2.303 \times 1.9872 \times 298.15 \times \log(2.9 \times 10^{-4})] = -65$ cal/mole

PROBLEM 7.23. **(a)** $\Delta H^\circ = -101.71 + 0 - (-101.68) = -0.030$ kcal/mole

$= -30$ cal/mole; $\Delta S^\circ = 22 - 39 = -17$ cal/deg mole

$$\ln K = \frac{\Delta S^\circ}{R} - \frac{\Delta H^\circ}{RT} = \frac{-17}{1.9872} - \frac{-30}{(1.9872)(298.15)} = -8.50412$$

$K_a = \exp(-8.50412) = 2.026 \times 10^{-4}$; $pK_a = 3.69$

(b) $\Delta G^\circ = -83.9 - (-89) = 5.1$ kcal/mole or 5100 cal/mole;

$$\ln K = -\frac{\Delta G^\circ}{RT} = -\frac{5100}{1.9872 \times 298.15} = -8.6078; K = 1.83 \times 10^{-4} \text{ M}; pK_a = 3.74$$

PROBLEM 7.24. (a) Using equation (13-77),

$$\% \text{ ionized acid} = \frac{100}{1 + antilog\ (7.47 - 5.83)} = 2.24\ \%$$

(b) $\Delta G^\circ = -RT \ln K_a = -1.9872 \times 298.15\ (-17.19985) = 10,191$ cal/mole

(c) 2.24% of 0.073 is 0.00164 M = $[A^-]$. The calculations are analogous to those in problem 7.22.

$$Q = \frac{(0.00164)^2}{(0.073 - 0.00164)} = 3.769 \times 10^{-5}$$

$$\Delta G = \Delta G^\circ + RT \ln Q = 10,191 + (1.9872)(298.15) \ln(3.769 \times 10^{-5})$$

$$\Delta G = 4156 \text{ cal/mole}$$

PROBLEM 7.25. For the first stage,

$\Delta H^\circ = -311.3 - (-308.2) = -3.1$ kcal/mole $= -3100$ cal/mole

$\Delta S^\circ = 21.3 - 42.1 = -20.8$ cal/deg mole

$$\ln K_1 = \frac{-20.8}{1.9872} - \frac{-3100}{1.9872 \times 298.15} = -5.234777$$

$$K_1 = 5.3 \times 10^{-3}; pK_1 = 2.27$$

For the second stage,

$\Delta H^\circ = -310.4 - (-311.3) = 0.9$ kcal/mole $= 900$ cal/mole

$\Delta S^\circ = -8.6 - 21.3 = -29.9$ cal/deg mole

$$\ln K_2 = \frac{-29.9}{1.9872} - \frac{900}{1.9872 \times 298.15} = -16.5653\ ; K_1 = 6.39 \times 10^{-8}; pK_2 = 7.19$$

For the third stage,

$\Delta H^\circ = -306.9 - (-310.4) = 3.5$ kcal/mole $= 3500$ cal/mole

$\Delta S^\circ = -52 - (-8.6) = -43.4$ cal/deg mole

$$\ln K_3 = \frac{-43.4}{1.9872} - \frac{3500}{1.9872 \times 298.15} = -27.7471$$

$K_3 = 8.9 \times 10^{-13}$; $pK_3 = 12.05$

Compare your results with those in Table 7 – 1 and in a handbook of chemical data.

PROBLEM 7.26. (a) $\Delta G^\circ = -271.3 - 56.79 - (-274.2 - 56.79) = 2.90$

kcal/mole = 2900 cal/mole ; $\ln K_1 = -\dfrac{\Delta G^\circ}{RT} = \dfrac{-2900}{1.9872 \times 298.15} = -4.89465$;

$K_1 = 7.49 \times 10^{-3}$; $pK_1 = 2.13$

(b) $\Delta G^\circ = 2.303 \, RT \, pK_2 = (2.303)(1.9872)(298.15)(7.21) = 9838$ cal/mole

or 9.84 kcal/mole

PROBLEM 7.27. (a) The reaction proceeds to the right, maintaining the value of the equilibrium constant, K.

(b) This reaction also proceeds to the right so as to maintain the value of K.

(c) $\Delta G^\circ = [-171.444 - 94.254 - 56.687] - [-241.9 - 2(-31.372)]$

$= -17.741$ kcal/mole $= -17741$ cal/mole ;

$\ln K = -\dfrac{\Delta G^\circ}{RT} = 29.94344$; $K = 1.01 \times 10^{13}$

PROBLEM 7.28. (a)

$\Delta G^\circ = [-171.444 - 56.687] - [-136.10 - 2(-31.372)] = -29.287$ kcal/mole

(b) $\ln K = -\dfrac{\Delta G^\circ}{RT} = 49.4308$; $K = 2.93 \times 10^{21}$

(c) $\Delta H^\circ = [-68.315 - 191.48] - [-143.81 - 2(39.952)] = -36.081$ kcal/mole

$\Delta S^\circ = [16.71 - 6.117] - [6.380 + 2(13.50)] = -22.787$ cal/deg mole

$\ln K = -\dfrac{\Delta H^\circ}{RT} + \dfrac{\Delta S^\circ}{R} = \dfrac{36081}{1.9872 \times 298.15} - \dfrac{22.787}{1.9872} = 49.4310$;

$K = 2.93 \times 10^{21}$. We obtain the same value for K as under **(b)**.

(d) ΔG° and K values are not changed. Adding or removing material only will change the direction of the reaction. The pH of the stomach fluid will increase with each tablet added.

PROBLEM 7.29. (a) The standard free energy is calculated from

$\Delta G^\circ = 2.303 \, RT \cdot pK_a$. For example, at 25° and 0.083 mole fraction of dioxane,

$\Delta G^\circ = 2.303 \times 1.9872 \times 298.15 \times 6.75 = 9210$ cal/mole

Table P7 – 1 for Problem 7.29

Mole fraction of dioxane, X_2							
	0.083		0.123		0.147		0.175
°C	25 35		25 35		25 35		25 35
$\Delta G°$ kcal/mole	9.2 9.2		9.9 9.9		10.2 10.2		10.6 10.6
$\Delta H°$ kcal/mole	10.5		10.1		9.7		10.1
$\Delta S°$ cal/°K mole	4.4 4.4		0.7 0.7		−1.6 −1.6		−1.6 −1.6

At 35°C and 0.083 mole fraction of dioxane,

$\Delta G° = 2.303 \times 1.9872 \times 308.15 \times 6.50 = 9167$ cal/mole

The results are shown in Table P7 – 1.

The standard enthalpy is obtained by integrating the van't Hoff equation for the two temperatures, T_1 and T_2:

$$\log K_2 - \log K_1 = \frac{\Delta H°(T_2 - T_1)}{2.303 \times R\, T_1 T_2}; \text{ since } pK_a = -\log K_a$$

$$-pK_{a2} + pK_{a1} = \frac{\Delta H°(T_2 - T_1)}{2.303 \times R\, T_1 T_2} \text{ and } \Delta H° = \frac{2.303 \times R\, T_1 T_2 (pK_{a_1} - pK_{a_2})}{T_2 - T_1}$$

For example, for 0.083 mole fraction of dioxane

$$\Delta H° = \frac{2.303 \times 1.9872 \times 298.15 \times 308.15 (6.75 - 6.50)}{308.15 - 298.15} = 10512 \text{ cal/mole}$$

The standard entropy is calculated from $\Delta G°$ and $\Delta H°$, according to the equation

$\Delta S° = \dfrac{\Delta H° - \Delta G°}{T}$. For example, at 35°C and 0.083 mole fraction of dioxane,

$$\Delta S° = \frac{10512 - 9167}{308.15} = 4.36 \text{ cal/deg mole}$$

The results for $\Delta G°$, $\Delta H°$, and $\Delta S°$ for all cases are shown in Table P7 – 1.

The reaction is not spontaneous since $\Delta G°$ is positive; however, this means that the process is not spontaneous in its standard state. The reaction does occur if ΔG (rather than $\Delta G°$) is negative, i.e., when the reaction quotient Q is less than K.

(b) By extrapolation, pK_a = 5.87 at 25° and 5.58 at 35°C (Figure P7 – 1)

Note that pK_a increases as the dielectric constant is lowered by addition of dioxane. That is, the dissociation constat K_a becomes smaller and the drug ionizes to a lesser extent as the dielectric constant decreases.

(c) Using linear regression in which X_2 (mole fraction of dioxane) is the independent variable,

At 25°C, pK_a = 10.81 X_2 + 5.87 ;

for X_2 = 0, pK_a = 5.87

At 35°C, pK_a = 10.95 X_2 + 5.61 ;

for X_2 = 0, pK_a = 5.61

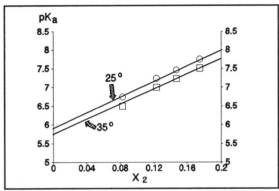

Figure P7-1 for Problem 7.29

PROBLEM 7.30. (a)

$\Delta G°$ = 2.303 RT pK_a

= (2.303)(1.9872)(293.15)(8.06)

= 10813 cal/mole

(b) $\Delta H°$ = $\Delta G°$ + T $\Delta S°$ = 10813 + (293.15)(– 3.1) = 9904 cal/mole

PROBLEM 7.31. K_a for acetic acid is 1.75 x 10^{-5} M (Table 7 – 1) ; ln K_a = – 10.9533

$\Delta G°$ = – RT ln K_a = – (1.9872)(298.15)(– 10.9533) = 6490 cal/mole

$\Delta S° = \dfrac{\Delta H° - \Delta G°}{T} = \dfrac{-92 - 6490}{298.15} = -22$ cal/(mole deg)

PROBLEM 7.32. (a) $\Delta G° = \frac{1}{2}(-50.35) - (\frac{1}{2} \times 0) - 0 = -25.175$ kcal/mole

(b) $\Delta H° = \frac{1}{2}(-63.32) - (\frac{1}{2} \times 0) - 0 = -31.66$ kcal/mole

$\Delta S° = \frac{1}{2}(46.8) - [\frac{1}{2}(53.286) + 18.5] = -21.74$ cal/deg mole

$\Delta G° = \Delta H° - T \Delta S° = -31660 - (298.15)(-21.74) = -25,177$ cal/mole

(c) Using the value obtained in part (a),

ln K = $\dfrac{-\Delta G°}{RT} = \dfrac{25,175}{(1.9872)(298.15)} = 42.4906$; K = 2.84 x 10^{18}

(d) The negative value of $\Delta G°$ indicates that the process is spontaneous in the standard state.

PROBLEM 7.33. (a) $\Delta G^\circ = (-79.70 - 56.690) - (-93.8 - 41.77)$
$= -0.82$ kcal/mole $= -820$ cal/mole

$$\ln K = \frac{-\Delta G^\circ}{RT} = \frac{820}{1.9872 \times 298.15} = 1.3840; \quad K = 3.99$$

(b) $\Delta H^\circ = (-114.49 - 68.317) - (-116.4 - 66.20) = -0.207$ kcal/mole
$= -207$ cal/mole

$\Delta S^\circ = 62.0 + 16.716 - (38.2 + 38.4) = 2.116$ cal/deg mole

$\Delta G^\circ = -207 - (298.15)(2.116) = -837.9$ cal/mole

$$\ln K = \frac{-\Delta G_o}{RT} = \frac{837.9}{1.9872 \times 298.15} = 1.4142; \quad K = 4.11$$

(c) $K = \dfrac{x \cdot x}{(0.0027 - x)(0.0027 - x)} = 4;$ $x = 0.0018$. The concentration of ethyl

acetate at equilibrium is 0.0018 mole/liter. An equal concentration, 0.0018 M of water is formed. The concentration of acetic acid and ethyl alcohol is therefore each 0.0027 − 0.0018, or 0.0009 M.

PROBLEM 7.34. (a) At 25°, $\Delta H^\circ = -116.843 - (-116.743)$
$= -0.1$ kcal/mole or -100 cal/mole

Knowing ΔH° and K_a at 25°C, the K_a value at 0°C is computed from the van't Hoff equation:

$$\ln \frac{K_2}{K_1} = \frac{\Delta H^\circ}{R}\left(\frac{T_2 - T_1}{T_1 T_2}\right)$$

K_2 at 25°C is 1.75×10^{-5}, $T_2 = 25 + 273.15 = 298.15°$K.
K_1 is obtained at 0°C using $T_1 = 0 + 273.15 = 273.15°$K and the van't Hoff equation:

$$\ln(1.75 \times 10^{-5}) - \ln K_1 = \frac{-100}{1.9872}\left(\frac{298.15 - 273.15}{273.15 \times 298.15}\right) = -0.01545$$

$\ln K_1 = 0.01545 + \ln(1.75 \times 10^{-5}) = -10.9379$; K_1 at 0°C $= 1.777 \times 10^{-5}$
At 37°C ($T_2 = 310.15$, $T_1 = 298.15$)

$$\ln K_2 \, (37°) - \ln K_1 \, (25°) = -\frac{100}{1.9872}\left(\frac{310.15 - 298.15}{298.15 \times 310.15}\right)$$

$\ln K_2 \, (37°) - \ln (1.75 \times 10^{-5}) = -0.006530;$ $\ln K_2 = -10.9598$ and $K_2 = 1.739 \times 10^{-5}$

(b) The CRC Handbook of Physics and Chemistry, 1st student ed., 1988, p. D − 103, gives the dissociation constant of acetic acid at several temperatures. Using these data, Figure P7 − 2 shows a plot of $\ln K_a$ against $1/T$ in the temperature range of 0° to 50°C. The relationship is not linear and $\ln K_a$ shows a maximum at 25°C. The Figure also shows the straight line and extrapolated values obtained above at 25° and 0° using the van't Hoff equation. This equation predicts a linear relationship between $\ln K_a$ and $1/T$ (solid straight line).

The extrapolated values obtained above are K_a = 1.739×10^{-5} at 37°C and 1.777×10^{-5} M at 0°C, respectively. Reading off from the curve of experimental values, K_a at 37°C and 0°C are 1.71×10^{-5} and 1.657×10^{-5}. Therefore, we cannot obtain accurate values by extrapolation when a curved line for $\ln K_a$ versus $1/T$ occurs.

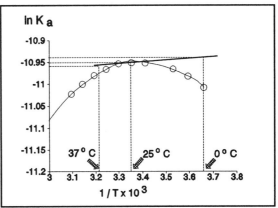

Figure 7-2 for Problem 7.34

PROBLEM 7.35. **(a)** At 35°C,

$$pK_a = \frac{\Delta G_o}{2.303\, RT} = \frac{10,260}{2.303 \times 1.9872 \times 308.15} = 7.28 \text{ at } 35°C$$

(b) We first compute $\Delta S°$ at 35° (assuming that $\Delta H°$ is constant in the temperature range of $20° - 35°$, $\Delta H° = 19320$ cal/mole):

$$\Delta S° = \frac{\Delta H° - \Delta G°}{T} = \frac{19320 - 10260}{308.15} = 29.4 \text{ cal/(deg mole)}$$

From the free energy and entropy at 35°C the pK_a at 20°C is obtained:

$$pK_a = \frac{10260 - 29.4(308.15 - 293.15)}{2.303 \times 1.9872 \times 293.15} = 7.32 \text{ at } 20°C$$

PROBLEM 7.36. 1 g in 500 ml = 2 g/liter or 2g/(165.23 g/mole) = 0.0121 molar

$[H^+] = -$antilog $(10.70) = 1.995 \times 10^{-11}$

At pH 10.70, $[OH^-] = \dfrac{K_w}{[H^+]} = \dfrac{10^{-14}}{1.995 \times 10^{-11}} = 5.012 \times 10^{-4}$

From equation $(7-24)$, $[OH^-] = \sqrt{K_b C_b}$;

$$K_b = \frac{[OH^-]^2}{C_b} = \frac{(5.012 \times 10^{-4})^2}{0.0121} = 2.0760 \times 10^{-5}; \quad pK_b = 4.68$$

PROBLEM 7.37. $[OH^-] = \sqrt{K_b C_b} = \sqrt{(7.6 \times 10^{-7})(0.01)} = 8.718 \times 10^{-5}$

$$a = \frac{[OH^-]}{C_b} = \frac{8.718 \times 10^{-5}}{0.01} = 0.0087 \text{ or } 0.87\%$$

Equation $(13-78)$ can also be used to calculate the percent of ionized species:

$$\% \text{ ionized} = \frac{100}{1 + antilog \ (pH - pK_a)} = \frac{100}{1 + antilog \ (9.94 - 7.88)} = 0.86 \ \%$$

where $pH = 14 - pOH = 14 - 4.06 = 9.94$

PROBLEM 7.38. (a) $\quad$ 3% solution $= \dfrac{30 \ g/\ell}{356.38 \ g/mole} = 0.0842 \ M$

$$[OH^-] = \sqrt{\frac{K_w \ C}{K_a}} = \sqrt{\frac{10^{-14} \times 0.0842}{1.74 \times 10^{-3}}} = 6.96 \times 10^{-7}$$

$$[H^+] = \frac{K_w}{[OH^-]} = \frac{10^{-14}}{6.96 \times 10^{-7}} = 1.4 \times 10^{-8} \ ; \ pH = 7.84$$

(b) The ionic strength of 0.9 g % of NaCl is equal to its molarity,

$$\mu = \frac{9 \ g/\ell}{58.45 \ g/mole} = 0.15398$$

The ionic strength of benzylpenicillin is its molarity, $\mu = 0.0842$
Total ionic strength, $\mu = 0.15398 + 0.0842 = 0.23818$

$$\log \gamma_\pm = \frac{-0.51 \ (1)^2 \sqrt{0.23818}}{1 + \sqrt{0.23818}} = -0.16727; \quad \gamma_\pm = 0.680$$

$$pH = \frac{1}{2} pK_w + \frac{1}{2} pK_a + \frac{1}{2} \log C + \log \gamma_\pm =$$

$$7.00 + \frac{1}{2}(2.76) + \frac{1}{2}\log(0.0842) + (-0.16727) = 7.68$$

PROBLEM 7.39. (a) $\quad$ 0.1 g/608 (g/mole) = 0.000164 (molarity)

$$[OH^-] = \sqrt{K_b C_b} = \sqrt{(4 \times 10^{-8}) \ (1.64 \times 10^{-4})} = 2.56 \times 10^{-6} \ M$$

(b) $\quad$ 9 g NaCl/1000 ml is 9 g/58.45 (g/mole) = 0.15398 molar NaCl = μ

$$\log \gamma_\pm = \frac{-0.51 \ (1)^2 \sqrt{0.15398}}{1 + \sqrt{0.15398}} = -0.14373; \ \gamma_\pm = 0.718$$

$$a_\pm = [OH^-] \gamma_\pm = (2.56 \times 10^{-6})(0.718) = 1.84 \times 10^{-6}$$

PROBLEM 7.40. (a) $\quad$ Figure P7$-$3 shows a plot of pK_a against δ_{OH}
(b) The equation obtained using least squares is:
$pK_a = 29.92 - 1.71 \delta_{OH}; \ r^2 = 0.967, \ n = 9$
(c) The pK_a of acetophenone oxime, as calculated from the equation is:
$pK_a = 29.92 - (1.71 \times 11.15) = 10.85$

Table P7 – 2 for Problem 7.41.

	pK$_a$	
Compound	Calculated	Literature
Benzaldehyde oxime	10.81	10.78
2,3 – Butanedione monooxime	9.13	9.34
Phenol	9.88	9.97
2 – Nitrophenol	7.42	7.14

PROBLEM 7.41. For benzaldehyde oxime, δ_{OH} = 11.19, pK$_a$ = 28.15 − (1.55 × 11.19) − (3.96 × 0) = 10.81
For phenol, δ_{OH} = 9.23, pK$_a$ = 28.15 − (1.55 × 9.23) − (3.96 × 1) = 9.88.
The results are given in Table P7 – 2.
The data are plotted in Figure P7 – 4.

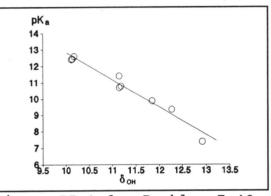

Figure P7-3 for Problem 7.40

PROBLEM 7.42.

$$T_{max} = \sqrt{\frac{A}{C}} = \sqrt{\frac{2324.47}{0.011856}}$$

= 442.78 °C

pK$_{Tmax}$ = $2\sqrt{AC}$ − D = (2 × 5.25) − 3.3491 = 7.15

ΔG° = 2.303(1.9872)[2324.47 − (3.3491 × 310.15) + (0.011856 × (310.15)^2]
= 11,103.61 cal/mole or 11.10 kcal/mole

ΔH° = 2.303(1.9872)[2324.47 − (0.011856 × (310.15)^2] = 5418.6 cal/mole or 5.42 kcal/mole

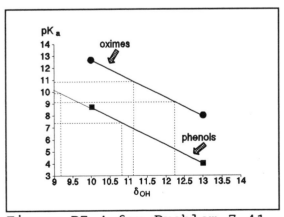

Figure P7-4 for Problem 7.41

ΔS° = 2.303(1.9872)[3.3491 − 2(0.011856)(310.15)] = −18.33 cal/mole deg

PROBLEM 7.43. The constants for lactic acid are A = 1304.72, C = 0.014926 and D = 4.9639 ;

$$T_{max} = \sqrt{\frac{A}{C}} = \sqrt{\frac{1304.72}{0.014926}} = 295.66^\circ K = 22.51^\circ C$$

$pK_{Tmax} = 2\sqrt{AC} - D = 8.8259 - 4.9639 = 3.862$

ΔG° = 2.303(1.9872)(A − DT + CT^2) = (2.303)(1.9872)[1304.72 − (4.9639)(298.15) + (0.014926)(298.15)^2] = 5270 cal/mole

ΔH° = 2.303(1.9872)(A − CT^2) = (2.303)(1.9872)[1304.72 − (0.014926)(298.15)^2] = −101 cal/mole

ΔS° = 2.303(1.9872)(D − 2CT) = (2.303)(1.9872)[4.9639 − (2)(0.014926)(298.15)] = −18 cal/mole deg

CHAPTER 8
Buffered and Isotonic Solutions

PROBLEM 8.1. $pH = pK_a + \log\dfrac{[salt]}{[acid]}$; $\log\dfrac{[salt]}{[acid]} = 8.8 - 9.24 = -0.44$;

$\dfrac{[salt]}{[acid]} = 0.363$. The ratio acid:salt is 1:0.36

PROBLEM 8.2.

$$pH = pK_w - pK_b + \log\frac{[base]}{[salt]} = 14 - 4.64 + \log\frac{0.10}{0.01} = 10.36$$

PROBLEM 8.3. (a)

$$pH = pK_a + \log\frac{[Na_2HPO_4]}{[NaH_2PO_4]} = 7.21 + \log\frac{[0.08]}{[0.12]} = 7.03$$

(b) Considering the ionic strength, for 0.08 M Na_2HPO_4,

$[Na^+] = 0.08 \times 2$ and $[HPO_4^{2-}] = 0.08$

For 0.12 M NaH_2PO_4,

$[Na^+] = 0.12$ and $[H_2PO_4^-] = 0.12$

$\mu = \dfrac{1}{2}[(0.08 \times 2 \times 1^2) + (0.08 \times 2^2) + (0.12 \times 1^2) + (0.12 \times 1^2)] = 0.36$

$$pH = 7.21 + \log\frac{0.08}{0.12} - \frac{0.51 \times 3\sqrt{0.36}}{1 + \sqrt{0.36}} = 6.46$$

PROBLEM 8.4. $pH = pK_a + \log\dfrac{[salt]}{[acid]} - \dfrac{0.51\sqrt{\mu}}{1 + \sqrt{\mu}}$

The ionic strenght, 0.20, is contributed by the 1:1 electrolyte, sulfisoxazole diethanolamine, in the concentration of 0.20 mole/liter.

$$pH = 5.30 + \log\frac{[0.20]}{[0.002]} - \frac{0.51\sqrt{0.20}}{1 + \sqrt{0.20}} = 7.14$$

PROBLEM 8.5. (a) 55 g/liter = 55/176.12 moles/liter = 0.312 M

$[H_3O^+] = \sqrt{K_a C_a} = \sqrt{(5\times10^{-5})(0.312)} = 3.95\times10^{-3}$

The assumptions that $C_a \gg K_2$, $[H_3O^+] \gg 2K_2$, and $C_a \gg [H_3O^+]$ are valid. Therefore equation (7−99) may be used, as done here, to calculate $[H_3O^+]$. One may then obtain the pH using the expression:

$$pH = -\log(3.95 \times 10^{-3}) = 2.40$$

(b) $pH = pK_a + \log \dfrac{[salt]}{[acid]}$; $\log \dfrac{[salt]}{[acid]} = 5.7 - 4.3 = 1.4$

The molar ratio [salt]/[acid] is 25.1 moles of sodium ascorbate and 1 mole of ascorbic acid (25.1:1)

$$\dfrac{25.1}{1 + 25.1} = 0.962 \text{ ; } 0.962 \times 100 = 96.2 \text{ \% of sodium ascorbate and } (100 - 96.2) =$$

3.8 % of ascorbic acid.

PROBLEM 8.6. **(a)** Physostigmine salicylate is a 1:1 salt of a weak acid and a weak base. Physostigmine's K_b is 7.6×10^{-7}. The K_a of salicylic acid is 1.06×10^{-3}. Equation $(7-127)$ and Example $7-22$ provide the necessary expressions to solve part **(a)**. From Table $7-2$, pK_a of the conjugate acid of physostigmine is 7.88; $K_a = 10^{-7.88} = 1.3 \times 10^{-8}$. Using equation $(7-127)$,

$$[H_3O^+] = \sqrt{K_1 K_2} = \sqrt{(1.06 \times 10^{-3})(1.3 \times 10^{-8})} = 3.71 \times 10^{-6} \text{ ; } pH = 5.43$$

where K_1 is the acidity constant for the acid (salicylic) and K_2 is the acidity constant for the conjugate acid of physostigmine. The assumptions are valid to allow the use of equation $(7-127)$.

(b) 0.5% = 5/413.5 moles/liter of physostigmine salicylate = 0.012 moles/liter

0.1 % = 1/275.34 moles/liter of physostigmine base (Table $7-9$) = 0.0036 mole/liter

$$pH = pK_w - pK_b + \log \dfrac{[base]}{[salt]} = 14 - 6.12 + \log \dfrac{0.0036}{0.012} = 7.36$$

Δ pH, increase = 7.36 - 5.43 = 1.93

PROBLEM 8.7. Since $\mu = 0.16$ and $pK_a = 6.33$,

$$pK' = pK - 0.51\sqrt{\mu} = 6.33 - 0.204 = 6.13$$

PROBLEM 8.8. The buffer capacity β is calculated from equation $(8-27)$:

$$\beta = 2.3\,C\dfrac{K_a[H_3O^+]}{(K_a + [H_3O^+])^2}. \text{ The unit on } \beta \text{ is mole/liter, but it is seldom shown.}$$

At pH 1, $\beta = 2.3 \times 0.2 \dfrac{(1.05 \times 10^{-4})(1 \times 10^{-1})}{[1.05 \times 10^{-4} + 1 \times 10^{-1}]^2} = 4.826 \times 10^{-4}$

Using the same kind of calculations for pH 2 through 7 the results are shown in Table P8 - 1 and are plotted in Figure P8 - 1.

Table P8 – 1 for Problem 8.8.

pH	1	2	3	4	5	6	7
ß	0.0005	0.005	0.039	0.115	0.0365	0.004	0.0004

The smooth line is obtained, calculating three additional points. From Figure P8 – 1, the maximum buffer capacity occurs at pH near 4. Using equation 8 – 17, we find:

$ß_{max}$ = 0.576 C = 0.576 x 0.2 = 0.1152 and it occurs at pH = pK_a = 3.98.

PROBLEM 8.9. For acetic acid, pK_a = 4.76 (Table 7 – 1). The pH of the solution is:

$$pH = pK_a + \log \frac{[salt]}{[acid]}$$

$$= 4.76 + \log \frac{[0.10]}{[0.20]} = 4.46$$

$[H_3O^+]$ = 3.47 x 10^{-5}

Using the Van Slyke equation, where K_a for acetic acid is 1.75 x 10^{-5},

$$\beta = 2.3 \times 0.3 \frac{(3.47 \times 10^{-5})(1.75 \times 10^{-5})}{[1.75 \times 10^{-5} + 3.47 \times 10^{-5}]^2} = 0.15$$

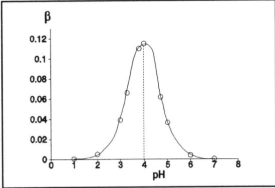

Figure P8-1 for Problem 8.8

PROBLEM 8.10. We chose NaH_2PO_4 as the acid and Na_2HPO_4 as the salt, where K_a of the acid is the second stage constant K_2 of phosphoric acid, 6.2 x 10^{-8}. We desire a buffer capacity ß = 0.10 at a pH of 6.5, i.e., at $[H_3O^+]$ = 3.162 x 10^{-7}. Using the Van Slyke equation and introducing C, the unknown total concentration, we have:

$$0.10 = 2.3 \, C \frac{(3.162 \times 10^{-7})(6.2 \times 10^{-8})}{[3.162 \times 10^{-7} + 6.2 \times 10^{-8}]^2}$$

Solving for C, we obtain C = 0.317, the total concentration of buffer. Now, using the Henderson – Hasselbalch equation with pK_a = 7.21 for the acid NaH_2PO_4, we compute the ratio, salt to acid

$$6.5 = 7.21 + \log \frac{[salt]}{[acid]} \; ; \; \log \frac{[salt]}{[acid]} = 6.5 - 7.21 = -0.71; \; \frac{[salt]}{[acid]} = 0.195$$

The total concentration is C = [salt] + [acid] = 0.317, and [salt] = 0.195[acid]. Therefore, [acid] + 0.195[acid] = 0.317, and [acid] = 0.265. Subtracting this value from the total concentration, [salt] = 0.317 – 0.265 = 0.052

The answer is Na_2HPO_4 (salt) = 0.052 M and NaH_2PO_4 (acid) = 0.265 M

PROBLEM 8.11. The initial pH is $3.75 + \log \dfrac{[0.1]}{[0.1]} = 3.75$

After adding 0.01 NaOH,

$$pH = 3.75 + \log \frac{0.1 + 0.01}{0.1 - 0.01} = 3.84; \quad \Delta pH = 3.84 - 3.75 = 0.09$$

$$\beta = \frac{\Delta base}{\Delta pH} = \frac{0.01}{0.09} = 0.111$$

If pH is not rounded to 3.84, one may obtain a somewhat different value, viz., ß = 0.115 instead of 0.111.

PROBLEM 8.12. At pH 7, $[H_3O^+] = 1 \times 10^{-7}$; K_a for boric acid is 5.8×10^{-10}. The buffer capacity is

$$\beta = 2.3 \times 0.36 \frac{(5.8 \times 10^{-10})(1 \times 10^{-7})}{[(5.8 \times 10^{-10}) + (1 \times 10^{-7})]^2} = 4.75 \times 10^{-3}$$

The same kind of calculations gives ß at the different pH values (Table P8 – 2).

The maximum buffer capacity is

$ß_{max} = 0.576C = 0.576 \times 0.36 = 0.207$. From Figure P8 – 2, this value occurs at pH 9.24, where pH = pK_a

Two additional points, not shown in Table P8 – 2 have been included in Figure P8 – 2.

The instructor should caution the students about the highly toxic nature of boric acid and its salts if taken internally. Boric acid could not be used systemically as a buffer.

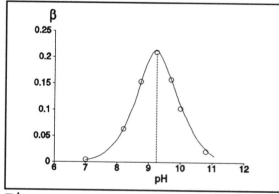

Figure P8-2 for Problem 8.12

Table P8 – 2 for Problem 8.12.

pH	7.0	8.2	9.24	10	10.8
ß	0.0047	0.064	0.210	0.103	0.021

PROBLEM 8.13. (a) At pH 5, $[H^+] = 1 \times 10^{-5}$,

$$\beta = 2.3 \times 0.067 \frac{(6.2 \times 10^{-8})\,(1 \times 10^{-5})}{[(6.2 \times 10^{-8}) + (1 \times 10^{-5})]^2} = 0.001$$

(b) At pH 7.2, $[H^+] = 6.31 \times 10^{-8}$

$$\beta = 2.3 \times 0.067 \frac{(6.2 \times 10^{-8})\,(6.31 \times 10^{-8})}{[(6.2 \times 10^{-8}) + (6.31 \times 10^{-8})]^2} = 0.04$$

PROBLEM 8.14. (a) The concentrations per liter are:

$$\frac{2.5\ g}{58.5\ g/mole} = 0.043 \text{ M sodium chloride}$$

$$\frac{2.8\ g}{381.43\ g/mole} = 7.3 \times 10^{-3} \text{ M sodium borate}$$

$$\frac{10.5\ g}{61.84\ g/mole} = 0.170 \text{ M boric acid}$$

The $-\log$ of the first dissociation constant, pK_1, of boric acid, from table $7-1$ is 9.24,

$$pH = 9.24 + \log \frac{7.3 \times 10^{-3}}{0.170} = 7.87$$

(b) The ionic strength of NaCl is equal to its molarity, $\mu = 0.043$. The concentration of $[H_3O^+] = [\text{borate}^-] = \text{antilog}(-7.87) = 1.35 \times 10^{-8}$. Its contribution to the total ionic strength can be disregarded: $\mu = 0.043 + (1.35 \times 10^{-8}) = 0.043$

$$pH = pK_a + \log \frac{[salt]}{[acid]} - \frac{0.51\ \sqrt{\mu}}{1 + \sqrt{\mu}}$$

$$pH = 9.24 + \log \frac{7.3 \times 10^{-3}}{0.170} - \frac{0.51\ \sqrt{0.043}}{1 + \sqrt{0.043}} = 7.79$$

PROBLEM 8.15. The equation for the buffer capacity of a strong electrolyte is:

$\beta = 2.303([H_3O^+] + [OH^-])$

For the strong base, NaOH, we have,

$[OH^-] = 3.0 \times 10^{-3}$, so $[H_3O^+] = \dfrac{K_w}{[OH^-]} = 3.3 \times 10^{-12}$

$\beta = 2.303(3.0 \times 10^{-3} + 3.3 \times 10^{-12}) = 0.0069$

PROBLEM 8.16. (a) Procaine + HCl $\rightarrow$ Procaine$^+$ + Cl$^-$

$$\text{Moles of procaine} = \frac{(0.1\ mole/\ell) \times 20\ ml}{1000\ ml/\ell} = 2 \times 10^{-3} \text{ mole}$$

Moles of HCl $= \dfrac{0.1 \times 10}{1000} = 1 \times 10^{-3}$ mole

Initial amount of procaine (base) $= 2 \times 10^{-3}$ mole
After neutralization with HCl:
$(2 \times 10^{-3}) - (1 \times 10^{-3}) = 1 \times 10^{-3}$ mole procaine base and salt is 1×10^{-3}. Thus the total amount of base + salt is $(1 \times 10^{-3}) + (1 \times 10^{-3})$ mole or 2×10^{-3} mole.
Mole of HCl = mole of procaine$^+$ (salt) $= 1 \times 10^{-3}$

$$pH = pK_w - pK_b + \log\frac{[base]}{[salt]} = 14 - 5.2 + \log\frac{1 \times 10^{-3}}{1 \times 10^{-3}} = 8.8$$

(b) Procaine hydrochloride, formed by the reaction of procaine base with HCl, yiels the total concentration, C:

$$\frac{2 \times 10^{-3}\ mole}{30\ ml} = \frac{C\ (mole)}{1000\ ml} \quad \text{or } C = 0.067 \text{ mole/liter}$$

At pH $= pK_a$, $\beta = \beta_{max}$, therefore we use the equation for the maximum buffer capacity,
$\beta_{max} = 0.576C = 0.576 \times 0.067 = 0.039$

PROBLEM 8.17. $\beta_{max} = (0.576)(0.026) = 0.015$
The maximum buffer capacity occurs when pH $= pK_a$, and the ratio of salt to acid $= 1$. The pH at which the maximum buffer capacity would occur is 6.1. The pK_a for carbonic acid at an ionic strength of 0.16 in the body is 6.1, not 6.37 as found in Table $7 - 1$.

PROBLEM 8.18. The pH of blood is 7.4, which is approximately equal to the pK_2 of phosphoric acid ($pK_2 = 7.21$), which corresponds to $K_2 = 6.2 \times 10^{-8}$. Therefore, we use a Na_2HPO_4/NaH_2PO_4 buffer.
We first calculate the total concentration required from the equation

$$\beta = 2.3\,C\frac{K_a\,[H_3O^+]}{(K_a + [H_3O^+])^2}$$

$$0.03 = 2.3\,C\,\frac{(6.2 \times 10^{-8})\,(3.98 \times 10^{-8})}{(6.2 \times 10^{-8} + 3.98 \times 10^{-8})^2}$$

Solving for C, the total concentration required is
$C = 5.48 \times 10^{-2}$ mole/liter
The ratio salt to acid is calculated from the Henderson – Hasselbalch equation, considering the ionic strength of blood, $\mu = 0.16$:

$$pH = pK_a + \log\frac{[salt]}{[acid]} - \frac{0.51\,(2Z - 1)\,\sqrt{\mu}}{1 + \sqrt{\mu}}\ ;$$

$$7.4 = 7.21 + \log\frac{[salt]}{[acid]} - \frac{0.51\times3\ \sqrt{0.16}}{1 + \sqrt{0.16}}\ ;$$

$$\log\frac{[salt]}{[acid]} = 0.6271;\qquad \frac{[salt]}{[acid]} = 4.24\ \text{or}\ \ [salt] = 4.24[acid].$$

We have calculated that the total concentration required is $C = 5.48 \times 10^{-2}$, therefore,

$5.48 \times 10^{-2} = [salt] + [acid] = 4.24[acid] + [acid] = 5.24[acid];$

$[acid] = 0.0105 = [H_2PO_4^-]$

$[salt] = 0.0548 - 0.0105 = 0.044 = [H_2PO_4^{2-}]$

Now, we calculate the ionic strength of this mixture,

$$\mu = \mu_{NaH_2PO_4} + \mu_{Na_2HPO_4} = \frac{1}{2}[(0.0105)(1)^2 + (0.0105)(1)^2 +$$

$$(0.044)(1)^2 + (0.044)(2)^2] = 0.12$$

We can prepare the buffer by using 0.011 M NaH_2PO_4 and 0.044 M Na_2HPO_4 and adding $(0.16 - 0.12) = 0.04$ M NaCl or KCl in order to adjust the ionic strength.

PROBLEM 8.19. (a) 50 ml x 0.2 N acetic acid (HAc) = 10 mEq (HAc)

10 ml x 0.2 N = 2 mEq NaOH in 60 ml;

10 − 2 = 8 mEq HAc in 60 ml (free acid)

The concentration of salt, sodium acetate is

$[salt] = \dfrac{2\ mEq\times1000}{60} = 33.33$ mEq/liter; the concentration of acid (HAc) is

$[acid] = \dfrac{8\ mEq\times1000}{60} = 133.33$ mEq/liter.

From the Henderson−Hasselbalch equation, the pH is

$$pH = 4.76 + \log\frac{33.33}{133.33} = 4.16$$

(b) 50 x 0.2 N (HAc) = 10 mEq of HAc

25 x 0.2 = 5 mEq NaOH; 10 − 5 = 5 mEq of HAc and 5 mEq sodium acetate.

$$pH = 4.76 + \log\frac{5}{5} = 4.76$$

(As shown in part **(a)**, the ratio [salt]/[acid] is independent of the volume, and in part **(b)** we can use the ratio 5/5 directly).

(c) 50 x 0.2 N (NaOH) = 10 mEq NaOH. Since we had initially 10 mEq HAc, the acid has been totally converted to salt, sodium acetate.

We therefore use the equation for a salt of a weak acid and a strong base to calculate the pH

$$pH = \frac{1}{2}pK_w - \frac{1}{2}pK_a + \frac{1}{2}\log c = 7 + 2.38 + \frac{1}{2}\log 0.1 = 8.88$$

where in the equation c is the molar concentration, ie., 10 mEq in 100 ml = 0.1 M

(d)   50.1 ml x 0.2 N NaOH = 10.02 mEq NaOH;

10.02 − 10 = 0.02 mEq NaOH in excess.

We have 10 mEq of sodium acetate. Its molarity is

$\dfrac{10 \times 10^{-3}}{100.1} = \dfrac{x}{1000}$; x = 0.0999 M sodium acetate. The molarity of NaOH is

$\dfrac{0.02 \times 10^{-3}}{100.1} = \dfrac{x}{1000}$; x = 1.998 x 10^{-4} M NaOH, $\dfrac{K_w}{K_a} = \dfrac{[HAc]\,[OH^-]}{[Ac^-]}$

Letting x = [HAc] and (x + 1.998 x 10^{-4}) = [OH$^-$],

$\dfrac{1 \times 10^{-14}}{1.75 \times 10^{-5}} = \dfrac{x(x + 1.998 \times 10^{-4})}{0.0999 - x}$;   solving for x,

$x = \dfrac{-3.50 \times 10^{-9} + \sqrt{(3.50 \times 10^{-9})^2 + 4\,(6.993 \times 10^{-20})}}{3.5 \times 10^{-5}} = 2.851 \times 10^{-7}$

[OH$^-$] = 2.851 x 10^{-7} + 1.998 x 10^{-4} = 2.0 x 10^{-4};

[H$_3$O$^+$] = $\dfrac{1 \times 10^{-14}}{2.0 \times 10^{-4}}$ = 0.5 x 10^{-10}; pH = 10.3.

PROBLEM 8.20. Assume 20 ml of 0.1 N barbituric acid,

$[H_3O^+] = \sqrt{K_a C_a} = \sqrt{(1.05 \times 10^{-4})\,(0.1)} = 3.24 \times 10^{-3}$;   pH = 2.49

Adding 5 ml NaOH, 5 x 0.1 = 0.5 base, 20 x 0.1 = 2; 2 − 0.5 = 1.5 acid left

$pH = pK_a + \log \dfrac{[salt]}{[acid]} = 3.98 + \log \dfrac{0.5}{1.5} = 3.50$

Using the same kind of calculations, the pH values after the addition of 10, 15, 20 and 21 ml NaOH are shown in the Table P8 − 3.

When we add 20 ml, we reach the equivalence point, and barbituric acid is totally converted to sodium barbiturate. We have 20 x 0.1 = 2 mEq sodium barbiturate in 40 ml, which is a 0.05 M solution.

$pH = \dfrac{1}{2}pK_w - \dfrac{1}{2}pK_a + \dfrac{1}{2}\log c = 7 + 1.99 + \dfrac{1}{2}\log 0.05 = 8.34$

Table P8 − 3 for Problem 8.20.

ml NaOH	5	10	15	20	21
pH	3.50	3.98	4.46	8.34	11.39

The pH at the equivalence point is 8.34 (see Table P8 – 3 and Figure P8 – 3).

Adding 21 ml NaOH, 21 X 0.1 = 2.1 mEq base; 2.1 − 2 = 0.1 mEq NaOH in excess in 41 ml solution.

$$\frac{0.1}{41} = \frac{x}{1000}; x = 2.439 \text{ mEq/liter} = 2.439$$

x 10^{-3} M [OH⁻]

pOH = 2.61 and pH = 14 − 2.61 = 11.39

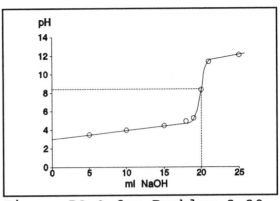

Figure P8-3 for Problem 8.20

(Table P8 – 3). Figure P8 – 3 shows the use of three additional points at 18, 19 and 25 ml NaOH to better complete the curve.

PROBLEM 8.21. 454.6 x 0.009 = 4.09 grains NaCl required

4.5 x 0.33 = 1.485 grain NaCl (equivalent to $AgNO_3$)

Therefore, 4.09 − 1.485 = 2.605 grain NaCl to be added

However, we want to add $NaNO_3$ since $NaCl \rightarrow AgCl \downarrow$

$$\frac{1\ NaNO_3}{0.68\ NaCl} = \frac{x}{2.605\ NaCl}; x = 3.83 \text{ grains or 248 mg } NaNO_3 \text{ to be added}$$

PROBLEM 8.22. Diphenhydramine is a 1:1 electrolyte

$$\Delta T_f = L_{iso} \times m = 3.4\ \frac{10}{291.81} = 0.12\ ; E = 17\ \frac{L_{iso}}{M} = \frac{17 \times 3.4}{291.81} = 0.20\ ;$$

V = 0.3 x 0.2 x 111 = 6.7 ml

PROBLEM 8.23. Using the Sprowls method,

V = 2.5 x 0.25 x 12.7 = 7.94 ml of solution required

The ml of solution required for isotonicity is greater than the volume of the solution to be prepared. This means that the quantity of ingredients in the solution produces a hypertonic solution. If only slightly hypertonic no adjustment need be made. If sufficiently hypertonic to cause irritation, the quantity of ingredients must be reduced to form an isotonic solution.

PROBLEM 8.24. (a) For sodium tetraborate, L_{iso} = 9.4. The compound's molecular weight is 381.43.

Molarity for isotonicity, M = $\dfrac{\Delta T_f}{L_{iso}} = \dfrac{0.52°}{9.4} = 0.0553$ mole/liter

Phenylephrine hydrochloride, L_{iso} = 3.5, m.w. = 203.67

$$M = \frac{0.52°}{3.5} = 0.149 \text{ mole/liter}$$

Physostigmine sulfate, L_{iso} = 5, m.w. = 648.45

$$M = \frac{0.52°}{5} = 0.104 \text{ mole/liter}$$

Calcium gluconate, L_{iso} = 4.2, m.w. = 448.39

$$M = \frac{0.52°}{4.2} = 0.124 \text{ mole/liter}$$

(b) For sodium tetraborate, 0.0553 mole/liter x 381.43 g/mole = 21.09 g/liter

$$\frac{21.09 \ g}{1000 \ ml \ H_2O} = \frac{0.3}{x}; x = 14.2 \text{ ml of water}$$

For phenylephrine hydrochloride, 0.149 mole/liter x 203.67 g/mole = 30.35 g/liter

$$\frac{30.35 \ g}{1000 \ ml \ H_2O} = \frac{0.3}{x}; x = 9.9 \text{ ml of water}$$

For physostigmine sulfate, 0.104 mole/liter x 648.45 g/mole = 67.44 g/liter,

$$\frac{67.44 \ g}{1000 \ ml \ H_2O} = \frac{0.3}{x}; x = 4.4 \text{ ml of water}$$

For calcium gluconate, 0.124 mole/liter x 448.39 g/mole = 55.60 g/liter

$$\frac{55.60 \ g}{1000 \ ml \ H_2O} = \frac{0.3}{x}; x = 5.4 \text{ ml of water}$$

PROBLEM 8.25.(a) Ascorbic acid:

For a 1% solution of NaCl, ΔT_f = 0.58°; the freezing point depression corresponding to 0.81% of NaCl required to get an isotonic solution of ascorbic acid can be computed from the proportion $\frac{1\%}{0.81\%} = \frac{0.58°}{x}; x = 0.47°$

Therefore the freezing point depression of the drug is the difference ΔT_f = 0.58° − 0.47° = 0.11°

Analogously, for the other drugs:

(b) Ephedrine sulfate:

$$\frac{1\%}{0.76\%} = \frac{0.58°}{x}; x = 0.44° ; \ \Delta T_f = 0.58° - 0.44° = 0.14°C$$

(c) Calcium chloride:

$$\frac{1\%}{0.48\%} = \frac{0.58°}{x}; x = 0.28°C ; \ \Delta T_f = 0.58° - 0.28° = 0.30°C$$

(d) Methacholine chloride:

$$\frac{1\%}{0.67\%} = \frac{0.58°}{x}; \; x = 0.39°C \; ; \; \Delta T_f = 0.58° - 0.39° = 0.19°C$$

PROBLEM 8.26. (a) $\quad E = 17 \dfrac{L_{iso}}{M}$

MgO is a di−divalent electrolyte, $L_{iso} = 2$, $E = 17 \dfrac{2.0}{40.3} = 0.84$

$ZnCl_2$ is a di−univalent electrolyte, $L_{iso} = 4.8$; $E = 17 \dfrac{4.8}{136.3} = 0.60$

$Al(OH)_3$ is a tri−univalent electrolyte, $L_{iso} = 6$; $E = 17 \dfrac{6}{77.98} = 1.31$

Isoniazid, a weak electrolyte, $L_{iso} = 2$; $E = 17 \dfrac{2}{137.2} = 0.25$

(b) Since E is the weight of NaCl with the same freezing point depression as 1 g of drug, from equation (8 − 43), $\quad \Delta T_f = 3.4 \dfrac{E}{58.54}$

in which 3.4 is the L_{iso} value for a 0.1 % solution of a 1:1 electrolyte (Table 8 − 3). Notice that

ΔT_f in equation (8 − 43) is for a 0.1 % solution, and we multiply by 10 to get $\Delta T_f^{1\%}$.

MgO, $\quad \Delta T_f = 3.4 \dfrac{0.84}{58.54} = 0.049°$. For a 1% solution, $\Delta T_f{}^{\%} = 0.49°$

The same result is obtained from the equation

$$\Delta T_f = L_{iso} \frac{1 \; g}{M} = 2 \frac{1}{40.3} = 0.049 \; °C \; or \; \Delta T_f^{1\%} = 0.49 \; °C$$

Analogously, for $ZnCl_2$,

$$\Delta T_f = 3.4 \frac{0.60}{58.45} = 0.035° \quad or \; \Delta T_f^{1\%} = 0.35°$$

$Al(OH)_3$, $\quad \Delta T_f = 3.4 \dfrac{1.31}{58.45} = 0.076° \quad or \; \Delta T_f^{1\%} = 0.76°$

Isoniazid, $\quad \Delta T_f = 3.4 \dfrac{0.25}{58.45} = 0.015° \quad or \; \Delta T_f^{1\%} = 0.15°$

PROBLEM 8.27. (a) From Table 10 − 4, E for tetracaine hydrochloride is 0.18, so 1 gram of drug is equivalent in terms of isotonicity to 0.18 gram of NaCl, and 10 gram of drug is equivalent to 10 x 0.18 = 1.8 gram NaCl. The total amount per liter of NaCl required for

isotonicity is 9 gram per 1000 ml, 9 − 1.8 = 7.2 gram of NaCl.
(b) E for boric acid is 0.50 from Table 8 − 4

$$\frac{1 \ g \ boric \ acid}{0.5 \ g \ NaCl} = \frac{x}{7.2 \ g \ NaCl}; \quad x = 14.4 \ g/\ell$$

The concentration in formula **(b)** is as in formula **(a)**. We just need boric acid to make 10 ml

of solution, therefore $\frac{14.4}{1000} = \frac{x}{10}$; x = 0.14 gram of boric acid.

PROBLEM 8.28. Chlorpromazine hydrochloride is a uni − univalent electrolyte,

L_{iso} = 3.4 (Table 8 − 3); E = 17 $\frac{3.4}{318.9}$ = 0.18

Na_2SO_4 is a uni − divalent electrolyte, L_{iso} = 4.3 ; E = 17 $\frac{4.3}{142.06}$ = 0.51

The E values for the other components are given in Table 8 − 4: E = 0.18 and 0.61 for
ascorbic acid and sodium bisulfite, respectively.
The volume of water necessary to make an isotonic solution is obtained as shown in Example
8 − 16: V = 111.1[(0.18 x 2.5) + (0.18 x 0.2) + (0.61 x 0.1) +
(0.51 x 0.1)] = 66.4 ml of water
We dissolve the drugs in 66.4 ml water (isotonic solution) and add (100 − 66.4) = 33.6 ml
of NaCl 0.9%, that is, 0.3 g of NaCl in 33.6 ml of water.

PROBLEM 8.29. L_{iso} = $\frac{0.52}{0.145}$ = 3.6; E = $\frac{17 \ L_{iso}}{M}$ = $\frac{17 \times 3.6}{300}$ = 0.20

V = w x E x 111, where w is the weight in grams of the drug.
V = (0.3)(0.20)(111) = 6.7 ml.

PROBLEM 8.30. 30 x 0.02 = 600 mg or 0.6 grams physostigmine.
0.600 x 0.16 = 0.096 g of NaCl equivalent to the mass of drug.
The isotonic NaCl solution contains 0.9 % NaCl;
Grams of NaCl required: 30 x 0.009 = 0.270
0.270 − 0.096 = 0.174 grams of NaCl to be added.

PROBLEM 8.31. Using the Henderson − Hasselbalch equation:

$\log \frac{[BH^+]}{[B]}$ = −pH + pK_w − pK_b = − 7.4 + 14 − 5 = 1.6;

$$\frac{[BH^+]}{[B]} = 39.8$$

$$\frac{39.8}{39.8 + 1} = 0.975 \text{ or } 97.5 \text{ % ionized drug;}$$

$100 - 97.5 = 2.5$ % nonionized drug.

The amount of aminophylline in the 10 – ml injectable is 0.25 grams or

$$\frac{0.25 \text{ } g}{421.2 \text{ } g/mole} = 5.9 \times 10^{-4} \text{ mole.}$$

The total molar concentration of aminophylline in blood is:

$$M = \frac{5.9 \times 10^{-4} \text{ } mole}{5 \text{ } \ell} = 1.2 \times 10^{-4} \text{ mole/liter}$$

The molar concentration of nonionized aminophylline is:

$1.2 \times 10^{-4} \times 0.025 = 3.0 \times 10^{-6}$ mole/liter.

CHAPTER 9
Electromotive Force and Oxidation – Reduction

PROBLEM 9.1. The Nernst equations for the individual electrodes are:

$$E_{Zn, Zn^{2+}} = E^o_{Zn, Zn^{2+}} - \frac{0.0592}{2} \log 0.2$$

$$E_{Cu^{2+}, Cu} = E^o_{Cu^{2+}, Cu} - \frac{0.0592}{2} \log \frac{1}{0.1}$$

$$E_{cell} = E_{Zn, Zn^{2+}} + E_{Cu^{2+}, Cu} = E^o_{Zn, Zn^{2+}} - \frac{0.0592}{2} \log 0.2 + E^o_{Cu^{2+}, Cu}$$

$$- \frac{0.0592}{2} \log \frac{1}{0.1} = E^o_{Zn, Zn^{2+}} + E^o_{Cu^{2+}, Cu} - \frac{0.0592}{2} \log \frac{0.2}{0.1} =$$

$$0.763 + 0.337 - \frac{0.0592}{2} \log 2 = 1.091 \text{ volt}$$

PROBLEM 9.2. The cell may be written

$$Cd| \ Cd^{2+} \ (a = 0.5)\| \ Ni^{2+} \ (a = 0.1)| \ Ni$$

We set up the cell so that oxidation takes place at the left electrode (the anode) and reduction at the right electrode (the cathode). From Table 9 – 1, the standard reduction potentials for cadmium and nickel are -0.403 and -0.230, respectively. Thus nickel is reduced more easily than cadmium, and the overall cell reaction is presumed to be

$$Cd + Ni^{2+} = Cd^{2+} + Ni$$

The Nernst equations for the individual electrodes are

$$E_{left} = E^o_{Cd, Cd^{2+}} - \frac{0.0592}{2} \log 0.5$$

$$E_{right} = E^o_{Ni^{2+}, Ni} - \frac{0.0592}{2} \log \frac{1}{0.1}$$

For the overall cell emf, we have

$$E_{cell} = E_{left} + E_{right} = (E^o_{Cd, Cd^{2+}} + E^o_{Ni^{2+}, Ni}) - \frac{0.0592}{2} \log \frac{0.5}{0.1}$$

$$= (+0.403) + (-0.230) - 0.0207 = 0.152.$$

Notice that the sign for $E^o_{Cd \rightarrow Cd^{2-}}$ was changed from the Table 9 – 1 value since oxidation rather than reduction is expected to occur if the Cd electrode is the anode. If we had made a mistake $E_{cell} = 0.152$ will be negative, and we must reverse the cadmium and nickel electrodes. However the sign of E_{cell} is positive, our presumptions are correct, and Ni is the cathode.

PROBLEM 9.3. The oxidation reaction (which is difficult to follow experimentally) is

$$Fe = Fe^{2+} + 2e$$

From equation (9 – 15), $\quad E_{electrode} = 0.440 - \dfrac{0.0592}{2} \log \dfrac{a_{Fe^{2+}}}{a_{Fe}}$

The activity of the ferrous ion, $a_{Fe^{2+}} = \gamma \times m = 0.40 \times 0.50 = 0.20$. Like all other pure solids and liquids, solid iron has an activity $a_{Fe} = 1$. Therefore

$$E_{electrode} = 0.440 - \dfrac{0.0592}{2} \log \dfrac{0.20}{1} = 0.461 \; volt$$

PROBLEM 9.4. $\quad E^{o}{}_{cell} = (E^{o}_{Fe,\,Fe^{2+}} + E^{o}_{Ni^{2+},\,Ni})$

$= (+0.440) + (-0.230) = 0.210$ volt

Emf of cell is

$$E_{cell} = 0.210 - \dfrac{0.0592}{2} \log \dfrac{0.2}{0.4} = 0.219 \; volt$$

PROBLEM 9.5. (a) The cell is written:

$$Li|\ Li^{+}\ (a = 1)\ \|\ Pb^{2+}\ (a = 1)|\ Pb$$

and the overall reaction is

$$Li + \tfrac{1}{2}Pb^{2+} = Li^{2+} + \tfrac{1}{2}Pb$$

(b) $\quad E^{o}_{cell} = (E^{o}_{Li \to Li^{+}} + E^{o}_{Pb^{2+} \to Pb}) = +3.045 - 0.126 = 2.919$

(c) $E_{cell} = E^{o}_{Pb,\,Pb^{2+}} + E^{o}_{Li^{+},\,Li} = (+0.126) + (-3.045) = -2.919$

Lead is more easily reduced, lithium is more easily oxidized. The reaction under **(c)** cannot occur. E_{cell} can never be negative.

PROBLEM 9.6. Here Zn is reduced and Cu is oxidized

$$E^{o}_{cell} = E^{o}_{\substack{left \\ oxid}} + E^{o}_{\substack{right \\ redn}} = E^{o}_{Cu \to Cu^{2+}} + E^{o}_{Zn^{2+} \to Zn} = -0.337 + (-0.763) = -1.100 \text{ volt}$$

We see that we mistakenly made Cu the oxidation electrode. The copper standard reduction potential $E^{o}_{Cu^{2+}/Cu}$ is $+0.337$, and $E^{o}_{Zn^{2+}/Zn}$ is -0.763, therefore Zn can reduce copper but copper cannot reduce zinc under standard conditions. The $E^{o}{}_{cell}$ voltage of -1.100 also indicates that zinc should be the left electrode and Cu the right electrode.

PROBLEM 9.7. (a) $Pt|\ H_2\ P(atm)|\ HCl\ (c,\ moles\ liter)|\ AgCl|\ Ag$

The individual reactions are:

$$\frac{1}{2}H_2 = H^+ + e^-$$

$$AgCl + e^- = Ag + Cl^-$$

The overal reaction is:

$$AgCl + \frac{1}{2}H_2 = H^+ + Ag + Cl^-$$

(b) From equation (9 − 18),

$$E = E^\circ - \frac{0.0592}{1}\ \log\ \frac{a_{H^+}a_{Ag}a_{Cl^-}}{a_{AgCl}a_{H_2}^{1/2}}$$

Since the solid phases are assigned an activity of 1 and the pressure of hydrogen gas is 1 atm, the equation becomes

$$E = E^\circ - \frac{0.0592}{1}\ \log\ a_{H^+}a_{Cl^-}$$

activity, $a_\pm = c\gamma_\pm = 0.50\ M \times 0.77 = 0.385$;

where $a_{H^+}a_{Cl^-} = a_\pm^2$

$E = 0.223 - 0.0592\ \log(0.385)^2 = 0.272$ volt

PROBLEM 9.8. The half cell potential E° for the mercury electrode is more positive than that of the iron electrode. Mercury is reduced more easily than iron and therefore cannot reduce the iron. If the cell is written as:

$$\frac{1}{2}Hg_2^{2+} + Fe^{3+} = Hg^{2+} + Fe^{2+},$$

$$E^\circ_{cell} = E^{\circ}_{(\frac{1}{2}Hg_2^{2+}\rightarrow Hg^{2+})} + E^{\circ}_{(Fe^{3+}\rightarrow Fe^{2+})} = -0.907 + 0.771 = -0.136$$

This result is wrong because E_{cell} cannot be negative.

PROBLEM 9.9. $E^\circ_{cell} = E^\circ_{left} + E^\circ_{right} = 0$

$$E_{cell} = 0 - \frac{0.0592}{2}\ \log\ \frac{0.023}{0.075} = 0.015\ volt$$

PROBLEM 9.10. (a) The free energy change for the cell reaction is

$\Delta G = -nFE = -1\ Eq/mole \times 96,500\ coul/Eq \times 0.361\ volt$

$= -34837\ J/mole$ or $-8326\ cal/mole$

(b) $\ln K = \dfrac{nFE^{\circ}}{RT} = \dfrac{-\Delta G^{\circ}}{RT} = \dfrac{1 \times 96500\ coul/mole \times 0.379\ volt}{8.314\ J^{\circ}K^{-1} \times 298.15^{\circ}K} = 14.75$

$K = \exp(14.75) = 2.55 \times 10^{6}$

$\Delta G^{\circ} = -RT \ln K = -(1.9872)(298.15)(\ln 2.55 \times 10^{6})$

$= -8740\ cal/mole = -36{,}568\ J/mole.$

PROBLEM 9.11. The Nernst equations are

$E_{left} = E^{o}_{Br^{-} \rightarrow AgBr} - \dfrac{0.0592}{1} \log a_1$

$E_{right} = E^{o}_{AgBr \rightarrow Br^{-}} - \dfrac{0.0592}{1} \log \dfrac{1}{a_1}$

Since E° is zero in a concentration cell,

$E_{cell} = E^{o}_{Br^{-} - AgBr} + E^{o}_{AgBr - Br^{-}} - 0.0592 \log \dfrac{0.02}{0.15}$

$E_{cell} = (-0.0592) \times (-0.8751) = 0.052\ volts$

PROBLEM 9.12. The half−cell reactions at anode and cathode are

$$Anode\ Zn = Zn^{2+}\ (m_1 = 0.01) + 2e$$
$$Cathode\ Zn^{2+}\ (m_2 = 0.1) = Zn$$

The activity coefficient $\gamma_{\pm}$ in the left half cell is 0.39 and in the right half cell is 0.15. The activities are therefore $a_1 = 0.01 \times 0.39 = 0.0039$ and $a_2 = 0.1 \times 0.15 = 0.015$. The overall reaction is

$$Zn^{2+}\ (a_1 = 0.0039) = Zn^{2+}\ (a_2 = 0.015)$$

The corresponding Nernst equation is

$E_{cell} = 0 - \dfrac{0.0592}{2} \log \dfrac{0.0039}{0.015} = 0.017$

PROBLEM 9.13. $\quad pH = pK_a - \dfrac{0.509\ Z^2 \sqrt{\mu}}{1 + a_i B \sqrt{\mu}} \quad$ *where* $\mu = 0.02$

$pK_a = 2.71 + \dfrac{0.509 \times 1\sqrt{0.02}}{1 + (3 \times 10^{-8})(0.33 \times 10^8)\sqrt{0.02}} = 2.773$

$K_a = 1.69 \times 10^{-3}$

PROBLEM 9.14. Using equation (9 – 44), where $\mu = 0.01$

$$pH = pK_a + \log\frac{[salt]}{[acid]} - \frac{AZ^2\sqrt{\mu}}{1 + a_iB\sqrt{\mu}}$$

$$7.66 = pK_a + \log\frac{0.01}{0.005} - \frac{0.509\,(1)^2\sqrt{0.01}}{1 + (2\times10^{-8})\,(0.33\times10^8)\,\sqrt{0.01}}$$

Solving for pK_a, one obtains $pK_a = 7.407$; $K_a = 3.92 \times 10^{-8}$

PROBLEM 9.15. $a_{H^+}a_{Br^-} = (\gamma_\pm c^2)$ and $E = E^\circ - 0.0592 \log(\gamma_\pm^2 c^2)$ (see equation 9 – 20);

$$\frac{0.4745 - 0.071}{-0.0592} = \log(\gamma_\pm^2) + \log(0.0004)^2$$

Solving for $\gamma_\pm$,

$$\log(\gamma_\pm^2) = -\log(0.0004)^2 + \frac{0.4745 - 0.071}{-0.0592} = -0.019998$$

$\text{antilog}(\gamma_\pm^2) = 0.955 = \gamma_\pm^2$; $\gamma_\pm = \sqrt{0.955} = 0.977$

PROBLEM 9.16. (a) $E_D = E^\circ - 0.03008 \log\frac{[Ox]}{[Rd]} + 0.06015\,pH$, since at 30°C

(303.15°K) , $\dfrac{2.303\,RT}{n\boldsymbol{F}} = \dfrac{2.303\times8.3143\times303.15}{2\times96,500} = 0.00030$

and for n = 1, $\dfrac{2.303\times8.3143\times303.15}{1\times96,500} = 0.06015$

We can also write $E_D = E^{\circ\prime} - 0.0296 \log\frac{[Ox]}{[Rd]}$, in which $E^{\circ\prime} = E^\circ - 0.06015\,pH$

In this solution of moderate acidity, we have

$E^{\circ\prime} = E_D + 0.03008 \log\dfrac{[Ox]}{[Rd]}$

$E^{\circ\prime} = -0.7850 + 0.03008 \log\dfrac{39.86}{60.14} = -0.790$ volt

(b) $E^{\circ\prime} = -0.8030 + 0.03008 \log\dfrac{71.5}{28.5} = -0.791$ volt

PROBLEM 9.17. We use 0.771 for the reduction electrode, i.e. $E_{Fe^{3+},\,Fe^{2+}} = 0.771$;

$E_D = 0.771 - \dfrac{0.0592}{1}\log\dfrac{10}{1} = 0.712$ volt

PROBLEM 9.18. $E^{o'} = +0.85$ at pH $= 0$

To get $E^{o'}$ at pH 8 we add $+0.0592 \log(1 \times 10^{-8})$ in which $1 \times 10^{-8} = a_{H^+}$;

$0.85 - 0.4736 = 0.3764 = E^{o'}$ at pH 8

$$\boldsymbol{E_D} = \boldsymbol{E^o} + 0.0592 \log a_{H^+} \pm \frac{0.0592}{n} \quad \text{where } n = 1. \text{ (See equations } 9 - 54 \text{ and } 9 - 55)$$

$$E_D = 0.3764 \pm 0.0592 = \begin{pmatrix} 0.436 & volt \\ 0.317 & volt \end{pmatrix}$$

PROBLEM 9.19. (a) $\quad E_D = E^{o'} - 0.03008 \log \frac{[Ox]}{[Rd]}$ at 30°C.

$$E^{o'} = -0.1284 + 0.03008 \log \frac{35.43}{64.57} = -0.1362 \text{ volt}$$

(b) $E^{o'} = -0.1670 + 0.03008 \log \frac{90.79}{9.21} = -0.1371 \text{ volt}$

(c) $\quad E^{o'}\text{(average)} = \frac{-0.1362 + (-0.1371)}{2} = -0.1367$

$$E^o = E^{o'}_{av.} + 0.06016 \text{ pH} = -0.1367 + (0.06016 \times 4.58) = 0.1388 \text{ volt}$$

PROBLEM 9.20. Each ml of 0.1 N potassium ferricyanide is equal to 0.87 mg of ascorbic acid in the orange juice.

If 6.8 ml of ferricyanide is needed to reach the endpoint of the titration, the concentration of ascorbic acid in 10 ml of orange juice is:

6.8 ml ferricyanide required in the titration times 0.87 mg ascorbic acid per ml of ferricyanide = mg of ascorbic acid in 10 ml of orange juice.

6.8 ml ferricyanide x $\dfrac{0.87 \; mg \; ascorbic \; acid}{ml \; ferricyanide}$ = 5.916/10 ml orange juice, or 59.2 mg

of ascorbic acid in 100 ml of orange juice.

PROBLEM 9.21. $E^o = E^{o'} + 0.06 \text{ pH} = -0.791 + 0.06(0.29) = -0.774 \text{ volt}$

PROBLEM 9.22. $\quad E_D = E^{o'} - \dfrac{0.0591}{2} \log \dfrac{[NADH]}{[NAD^+] \, [H^+]}$

$$E_D = -0.320 - 0.0296 \log \frac{1}{0.1} = -0.320 - (0.0296 \times 1) = -0.3496 \approx -0.350 \text{ volt}$$

PROBLEM 9.23. $E^{o\prime} = -0.197 - (-0.320) = +0.123$ volt

$$lnK = \frac{nFE^{o\prime}}{RT} = \frac{2(96500)(0.123)}{(8.314)(298.15)} = 9.5767$$

$K = e^{9.5767} = 1.44 \times 10^4$

$\Delta G^{o\prime} = -nFE^{o\prime} = -(2)(96500)(0.123) = -23739$ J/mole

or $\Delta G^{o\prime} = -RT \ln K = -(8.314)(298.15)(9.5816) = -23752$ J/mole or without rounding in each step one gets $\Delta G^{o\prime} = -23739$ J/mole or -5674 cal/mole.

CHAPTER 10
Solubility and Distribution Phenomena

PROBLEM 10.1. $1.80 \frac{mg}{ml} \times \frac{g}{10^3 mg} \times \frac{10^3 ml}{\ell} = 1.80$ g/liter

$$M = \frac{1.80 \ g/\ell}{280.32 \ g/mole} = 6.421 \times 10^{-3} \ M$$

(b)   1 liter of solution weights 1000 ml x 1.0086 g/ml = 1008.6 g

Grams of solvent = grams solution − grams of solute = 1008.6 − 1.80 = 1006.8 g

$$\frac{(1.80 \ g/280.32 \ g/mole)}{1006.8 \ g \ solvent} = \frac{x}{1000 \ g \ solvent}$$

x = molality = 6.378×10^{-3}

(c)   weight of dioxane in the 90:10 v/v mixture:

10 x 1.0313 = 10.313 g ; 10.313 g/(88.10 g/mole) = 0.1171 mole

weight of water in the 90:10 v/v mixture:

90 ml x 0.9970 = 89.73 g; 89.73 g/(18.015 g/mole) = 4.9808 mole

Total weight of the water − dioxane mixture:

10.313 g dioxane + 89.73 g water = 100.043 g

Moles of solute in the mixture:

Using the molality found in part **(b)**,

$$\frac{6.378 \times 10^{-3} \ mole \ solute}{1000 \ g \ solvent \ mix.} = \frac{x \ mole \ solute}{100.043 \ g \ solvent \ mix.} ;$$

x = 6.3807×10^{-4} mole of solute

The mole fraction is

$$X_2 = \frac{n_2}{n_1 + n_2 + n_3} = \frac{6.3807 \times 10^{-4}}{6.3807 \times 10^{-4} + 0.1171 + 4.9808} = 1.251 \times 10^{-4}$$

PROBLEM 10.2. $\frac{V_{gas}, STP}{V_{soln}} = \alpha p$; for CO_2, $\alpha = 0.759$ (Table 10.3)

$V_{gas} = 0.759$ atm^{-1}x 0.7 atm x 1 liter = 0.53 liter at STP

PROBLEM 10.3.   For oxygen in water at 25° and at a partial pressure of 610 mm Hg, c, the solubility of O_2 is: c = σ p = 5.38×10^{-5} g liter^{-1} mm^{-1} x 610 mm Hg

= 0.0328 g liter^{-1}

Note: σ is simply the reciprocal of k, the values of which are found in Table 10 − 4.

PROBLEM 10.4. $k_{He} = 1.99 \times 10^6$ torr/molality $= \dfrac{187.5 \; mm}{molality}$;

Molality $= 9.42 \times 10^{-5}$ moles/kg blood

Since the percent of He at saturation in the red blood cells is 85.5%,

Amount dissolved $= 0.855 \times 9.42 \times 10^{-5} = 8.06 \times 10^{-5}$ moles/kg blood.

PROBLEM 10.5. $X_2 = \dfrac{p}{k} = \dfrac{610}{6.51 \times 10^7} = 9.37 \times 10^{-6}$

$m = \dfrac{1000 X_2}{M_1 (1 - X_2)} = \dfrac{1000 \times 9.37 \times 10^{-6}}{18.015 (1 - 9.37 \times 10^{-6})} = 5.20 \times 10^{-4}$

PROBLEM 10.6. (a)   At a depth of 30 meters, h = 30 meters x 100 cm/meter = 3000 cm; $P = \rho g h = 1.0$ g/cm^3 x 980 cm sec^{-2} x 3000 cm $= 2.94 \times 10^6$ g cm/sec^2 = 2.94×10^6 dyne cm^{-2}.

To convert to atm,

2.94×10^6 dyne cm^{-2} x$\left(\dfrac{1 \; atm}{1.01325 \times 10^6 \; dyn \; cm^{-2}}\right)$ = 2.9016 atm or approximately 2.90

atm pressure at a depth of 30 meters in the lake. Add 1 atm for pressure in air to give the total pressure of P = 3.90 atm.

For the partial pressure of O_2 at this depth to be 0.2 atm we need the gas law, $P = \dfrac{nRT}{V}$.

For the fractional pressure of O_2,

P_{O_2}/P_{total} to equal 0.20 atm/3.90 atm we have

$$\dfrac{P_{O_2}}{P_{total}} = \dfrac{n_{O_2}(RT/V)}{n(RT/V}) = \dfrac{n_{O_2}}{n} = X_{O_2}$$

The volume fraction must equal the mole fraction, X_{O_2}, therefore

$X_{O_2} = \dfrac{0.20 \; atm}{3.90 \; atm} = 0.051$

or the percent by volume of O_2 in the mixture at this depth is 0.051 x 100 = 5.1%

(b)   P = 2.5 atm x 1.01325 x 10^6 dyne cm^{-2}/atm = 2.533125 x 10^6 dyne cm^{-2}

P = ρgh ; 2.533125 x 10^6 dyne cm^{-2} = 1.0 g/cm^3 x 980 cm/sec^2 x h;

h = 2584.8 cm or 25.85 meters.

(c)   If h = 50 m or 5000 cm,

P = 1.0 g/cm^3 x 980 cm/sec^2 x 5000 cm = 4.9 x 10^6 dyne cm^{-2};

4.9×10^6 dyne cm^{-2} x $\dfrac{1\ atm}{1.01325 \times 10^6\ dyn\ cm^{-2}}$ = $4.8\ atm$. This is the pressure

produced by the 50 meter depth of water. But overlaying the water of the lake is atmospheric air pressing down with a pressure of 1 atm. Therefore the pressure at a depth of 50 meters is 4.8 atm + 1 atm = 5.8 atm.

(d) The partial pressure of He in the mixture is 80/100 = 0.8. Using the Henry's law,

$X_2 = \dfrac{p}{k} = \dfrac{0.8\ atm}{1.45 \times 10^5\ (atm/mole\ fraction)}$ = 5.52×10^{-6}

(e) $X_2 = \dfrac{p}{k} = \dfrac{3.12\ atm}{1.45 \times 10^5\ (atm/mole\ fraction)}$ = 2.15×10^{-5}

(f) From part **(e)** we found the mole fraction solubility for He in the blood at a 30 meter depth in the lake to be $X_2 = 2.15 \times 10^{-5}$; M_1 of water = 18.015, we use the same for blood,

$m = \dfrac{1000\,X_2}{M_1\,(1 - X_2)} = \dfrac{1000 \times 2.15 \times 10^{-5}}{18.015\,(1 - 2.15 \times 10^{-5})}$ =

1.193×10^{-3} mole/kg blood.
The solubility of He in 6 kg of blood is
1.193×10^{-3} mole/kg blood x 6 kg blood = 0.00716 mole He in the blood of an adult.

(g) The body temperature is 37°C (310.15°K), P = 3.12 atm and from part **(f)** n = 0.00716 mole. Using the ideal gas equation, $V_2 = \dfrac{nRT}{P}$ =

$\dfrac{0.00716\ mole \times 0.0821\ (atm\ \ell/deg\ mole) \times 310.15\ deg}{3.12\ atm}$ = $0.0584\ \ell$

The volume of helium in 6 kg of blood is 0.0584 liter or 58.4 cm^3

(h) The solubility of He at the total pressure of 2.3 (pressure under the surface of the lake) + 1 (atmospheric pressure) = 3.3 atm, using Henry's law is

$X_2 = \dfrac{3.3 \times 0.8\ atm}{1.45 \times 10^5\ (atm/mole\ fraction)}$ = 1.82×10^{-5}

Note that we multiply the pressure by 0.8 because He is only 80%.
The number of moles, n, of He/kg blood is its molality, m:

$m = \dfrac{1000\,X_2}{M_1\,(1 - X_2)} = \dfrac{1000 \times 1.82 \times 10^{-5}}{18.015\,(1 - 1.82 \times 10^{-5})}$ = 0.0010 mole/(kg blood).

In 6 liters or kg's of blood, $0.0010 \times 6 = 6.0 \times 10^{-3}$ mole
Using the ideal gas equation,

$$V_2 = \frac{nRT}{P} = \frac{0.0060 \times 0.0821 \times 310.15}{3.3} = 0.0463 \text{ liter}$$

The volume of helium is 0.0463 liter or 46.3 cm^3

For a change from P_2 = 3.3 atm to P_1 = 1 atm, we have

$$\frac{V_1}{V_2} = \frac{P_2}{P_1}; \quad V_1 = 46.3 \text{ } cm^3 \frac{3.3 \text{ } atm}{1.0 \text{ } atm} = 152.8 \text{ } cm^3, \text{ and finally,}$$

$V_1 - V_2$ = 152.8 − 46.3 = 106.5 cm^3 of helium as bubbles in the blood.

PROBLEM 10.7. First, we convert % by weight to mole fraction,

$$X_2 = \frac{n_2}{n_1 + n_2}, \text{ in which n is the number of moles. For example, the mole fraction of 65 \%}$$

by weight of succinic acid is:

$$X_2 = \frac{65/118.09}{(65/118.09) + (35/352.8)} = 0.8473$$

Analogous calculations give the mole fraction of succinic acid (Table P10 − 1) and griseofulvin (Table P10 − 2) at the several temperatures, expressed in °C and °K.

Figure P10 − 1 shows the phase diagram, a plot of temperature (°C) against the mole fraction of succinic acid.

The intersection of the curves gives the eutectic point at 173°C, corresponding to a mixture of 0.70 succinic acid (read on the x − axis) and 0.30 griseofulvin (in mole fraction).

The melting point temperatures for the pure components are read on the vertical axis at X_2^i = 1.

For succinic acid, T_o = 187°C.

For griseofulvin, T_o = 219°C.

Using the ideal solubility expression in the form of a linear regression equation, we have for succinic acid (data from Table P10 − 1):

$$\ln X_2^i = -\frac{\Delta H_f}{R} \frac{1}{T} + \text{constant}$$

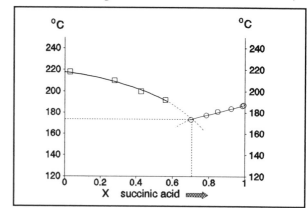

Figure P10-1 for Problem 10.7

$$-\ln X_2^i = -5239.233 \frac{1}{T} + 11.37710 \text{ ;}$$

r^2 = 0.9861

ΔH_f = 1.9872 x (−slope) = (1.9872)(5239.233) = 10,411 cal/mole.

Table P10 – 1 for Problem 10.7.

Succinic Acid			
T, °C (K°)	1/T x 10^3	X$_2$	ln X$_2$
187.2 (460.2)	2.173	0.9932	− 0.0068
186.6 (459.6)	2.176	0.9862	− 0.0139
183.8 (456.8)	2.189	0.9228	− 0.0804
181 (454)	2.197	0.8473	− 0.1657
177.6 (450.6)	2.219	0.7850	− 0.2405
173.3 (446.3)	2.240	0.7013	− 0.3549

Table P10 – 2 for Problem 10.7

Griseofulvin			
T, °C (°K)	1/T x 10^3	X$_2$	ln X$_2$
218 (491)	2.037	0.9707	− 0.0297
210 (483)	2.070	0.7508	− 0.02866
200 (473)	2.114	0.5724	− 0.05578
192 (465)	2.150	0.4385	− 0.8243

When $X_2^i = 1$, $\ln X_2^i = 0$,

$$0 = 5239.233 \frac{1}{T} + 11.3770$$

T = 460.4 °K = 187.3°C for the pure component (Merck Index gives 185° − 187°C).
For griseofulvin (data from Table P10 − 2) the equation is:

$$-\ln X_2^i = -6916.415 \frac{1}{T} + 14.0497; r^2 = 0.9981$$

ΔH_f = slope x 1.9872 = 6916.415 x 1.9872 = 13,744 cal/mole.

When $X_2 = 1$, $\ln X_2 = 0$, $0 = 6916.415 \frac{1}{T} + 14.0497$

T = 492.3 °K = 219.3°C (Merck Index gives 220°C)

PROBLEM 10.8.   Since the phenol-water system cannot have greater than 34% phenol at 65.85°C, the balance, 66% must be H_2O,

$1000 \times 0.66 = 660$ g H_2O, which equals the minimum % w/w of H_2O which can be present at 65.85°C and maintain only one phase.

PROBLEM 10.9.   The summation of the weight of the two phases, A (aqueous) and B (phenol) must equal the total weight, 200 g. Also, the summation of the weight of phenol in each phase must equal the total amount initially added,

$$200 = A + B$$
$$0.2(200) = 0.13A + 0.6B, \text{ or}$$
$$0.2(200) = 0.13A + 0.6(200 - A)$$

$80 = 0.47A$; $A = 170.2$ g. Since only 13% phenol is present, the amount of phenol in the aqueous phase is

$170.2 \times 0.13 = 22.13$ g phenol in phase A.

The phenol layer, B weighs

$$B = 200 - A = 200 - 170.2 = 29.8 \text{ g}$$

The weight of phenol in the phenol layer is

$29.8 \times 0.6 = 17.9$ g phenol in phase B.

PROBLEM 10.10.   For hexane, carbon 1 is connected by one bond to carbon 2, which is joined to its adjacent carbons by two bonds. For the first term in the $^1\chi$ equation we therefore write $(1 \times 2)^{-1/2}$. The fifth carbon follows the same rule and is also written $(1 \times 2)^{-1/2}$. Carbon 2 is connected by two bonds, one to carbon 1 and the other to carbon 3. Its term is therefore written $(2 \times 2)^{-1/2}$. Carbons 3 and 4 follow the same rule and are also written $(2 \times 2)^{-1/2}$.

$$
\begin{matrix}
\text{C} & & \text{C} & & \text{C} \\
& {}_1\diagdown \, {}^2 & & {}_4 \diagup & \\
& & {}_3 & & \\
& \text{C} & & \text{C} &
\end{matrix}
$$

$^1\chi = (1 \times 2)^{-1/2} + (2 \times 2)^{-1/2} + (2 \times 2)^{-1/2} + (2 \times 2)^{-1/2} + (1 \times 2)^{-1/2} = 2.914$;

$\ln S = -1.505 - 2.533\,^1\chi = -8.886162$; $S = 1.38 \times 10^{-4}$ mole/liter

PROBLEM 10.11. $\ln S = -0.0430(HYSA) - 0.0586(FGSA) + 8.003(I) + 4.420$

(a) Cyclohexanol, HYSA = 240.9, FGSA = 49.6, $I = 1$

$\ln S = -0.0430(240.9) - 0.0586(49.6) + 8.003(1) + 4.420 = -0.84226$;

$S = 0.431$ mole/(kg solvent) ;   % error $= \dfrac{0.38 - 0.431}{0.38} \times 100 = -13.4$ %

(b)   n–octane, HYSA = 383, FGSA = 0, I = 0,

ln S = (−0.0430)(383) − (0.0586)(0) + 0 + 4.420 = −12.049

S = 5.85 x 10^{-6} mole/(kg solvent);

% error = $\dfrac{5.80 \times 10^{-6} - 5.85 \times 10^{-6}}{5.80 \times 10^{-6}}$ = −0.86 %.

PROBLEM 10.12.   Polymorph form I:

$$\ln X_2^{\,i} = -\frac{\Delta H_f}{R}\left(\frac{T_f - T}{T_f T}\right) = -\frac{9550}{1.9872}\left(\frac{431 - 298}{431 \times 298}\right) = -4.9765$$

$$X_2^{\,i} = 0.0069$$

Polymorph II:

$$\ln X_2^{\,i} = -\frac{9700}{1.9872}\left(\frac{426 - 298}{426 \times 298}\right) = -4.9217;\quad X_2^{\,i} = 0.0073$$

Polymorph VII:

$$\ln X_2^{\,i} = -\frac{2340}{1.9872}\left(\frac{368 - 298}{368 \times 298}\right) = -0.7516;\quad X_2^{\,i} = 0.472$$

The ideal solubilities decrease in the following order: VII > II > I

The melting point are useful in ordering the ideal solubility of the polymorphs; the smaller the melting point, the larger the solubility. Note: Both o and f are used as subscripts on quantities such as ΔH and T to signify the value at its melting point.

PROBLEM 10.13.

$$\ln X_2^{\,i} = -\frac{\Delta H_f}{R}\left(\frac{T_f - T}{T_f T}\right) = -\frac{4139}{1.9872}\left(\frac{395.15 - 298.15}{395.15 \times 298.15}\right) = -1.7149$$

$$X_2^{\,i} = 0.180$$

PROBLEM 10.14.   Sulfamethoxypyridazine:

$$\ln X_2^{\,i} = -\frac{\Delta H_f}{R}\left(\frac{T_f - T}{T_f T}\right) = -\frac{8110}{1.9872}\left(\frac{453.55 - 298.15}{453.55 \times 298.15}\right) = -4.6900$$

$$X_2^{\,i} = 0.0092$$

Sulfameter:

$$\ln X_2^{\,i} = -\frac{9792}{1.9872}\left(\frac{484.75 - 298.15}{484.75 \times 298.15}\right) = -6.3620;\quad X_2^{\,i} = 0.0017$$

Sulfisomidine:

$$\ln X_2^{\,i} = -\frac{10781}{1.9872}\left(\frac{515.35 - 298.15}{515.35 \times 298.15}\right) = -7.6690;\quad X_2^{\,i} = 4.67 \times 10^{-4}$$

Table P10 − 3 for Problem 10.15.

1/T (°K $^{-1}$) x 10^3	ln X_2^i
2.911	−0.1744
2.963	−0.2984
3.150	−0.7298
3.252	−0.9365
3.367	−1.1744
3.503	−1.4610

Table P10 − 4 for Problem 10.15.

T (°K)	ΔH_f (cal/mole)
343.5	4249.6
337.5	4448.2
317.5	4532.7
307.5	4406.0
297.0	4343.1
285.5	4314.1

PROBLEM 10.15. (a) The data needed for regression analysis are shown in Table P10 − 3.

The regression equation is

$$\ln X_2 = -2169.07 \frac{1}{T_f} + 6.13;$$

$r^2 = 0.9992$

ΔH_f = (−slope) x 1.9872 = 2169.07 x 1.9872 = 4,310 cal/mole.

ΔS_f = intercept x 1.9872 = 6.13 x 1.9872 = 12.18 cal/mole deg

(b) Using equation $(10-11)$, ΔH_f at 343.5 °K is obtained as:

$$\Delta H_f = \frac{-\ln X_2^i \, R}{\left(\dfrac{T_f - T}{T_f T}\right)} = \frac{0.1744 \times 1.9872}{\left(\dfrac{353.4 - 343.5}{353.4 \times 343.5}\right)}$$

= 4249.6 cal/mole

Analogous calculations for the other temperatures give the results presented in Table 10P−4. The average of the six values above is $\Delta \overline{H_f}$ = 4382 cal/mole.

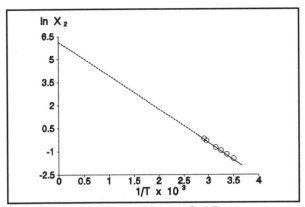

Figure P10-2 for Problem 10.15

Figure P10−2 shows the experimental points and the extrapolated values of $\ln X_2$ at $1/T = 0$, i.e., at $T = \infty$

PROBLEM 10.16.

$\ln X_2^i = \ln (0.179) = -1.7204$

$$\Delta H_f = \frac{-\ln X_2^i \times R}{\left(\dfrac{T_f - T}{T_f T}\right)} = \frac{1.7204 \times 1.9872}{\left(\dfrac{395.55 - 298.15}{395.55 \times 298.15}\right)} = 4144 \text{ cal/mole}$$

PROBLEM 10.17.
The molar heat of vaporization of ethyl acetate is

ΔH_v = 97.5 cal/g x·88.1 g/mole = 8589.75 cal/mole, and the molar volume is V = 88.1/0.9 = 97.89 cm³/mole

The solubility parameter of ethyl acetate is:

$$\delta = \left(\frac{\Delta H_v - RT}{V}\right)^{\frac{1}{2}} = \left(\frac{8589.75 - 1.9872 \times 298.15}{97.89}\right)^{\frac{1}{2}} = 9.0 \ (cal/ml)^{-1/2}$$

The ideal solubility of benzoic acid is calculated from:

$$\ln X_2^i = -\frac{\Delta H_f}{R}\left(\frac{T_f - T}{T_f T}\right) = \frac{-4135.8}{1.9872}\left(\frac{395.15 - 298.15}{395.15 \times 298.15}\right) = -1.7135$$

where ΔH_f = 33.9 cal/g x 122 g/mole = 4135.8 cal/mole. Taking the antilogarithm, the ideal solubility is X_2^i = 0.1802

Using the Hildebrand equation and assuming that $\varphi = 1$ for a first approximation,

$$-\ln X_2 = -\ln X_2^i + \frac{V_2 \phi_1^2}{RT}(\delta_1 - \delta_2)^2 =$$

Table P10 – 5 for Problem 10.18.

Solvent	Acetone	Hexane	Methanol	Acetic acid	Water	Chlorobenzene
γ_2	1.2	2.0	10.8	3.8	2.5×10^4	1.0

$$1.7135 + \frac{(104.4)(1)^2}{(1.9872)(298.15)}(11.3 - 9)^2 = 2.6456; \quad X_2 = 0.07096$$

For the second approximation, we use $\phi_1 = (1 - X_2) = 1 - 0.07096 = 0.92904$

$$-\ln X_2 = 1.7135 + \frac{(104.4)(0.92904)^2}{(1.9872)(298.15)}(11.3 - 9)^2 = 2.5180;$$

$X_2 = \exp(-2.5180) = 0.08062$.

Third approximation, $\phi_1 = (1 - 0.08062) = 0.91938$, the calculated X_2 value is 0.081970.

4th approximation, $\phi_1 = (1 - 0.081970) = 0.91803$; $X_2 = 0.081677$

5th approximation, $\phi_1 = (1 - 0.081677) = 0.918323$; $X_2 = 0.081636$

6th approximation, $\phi_1 = (1 - 0.081636) = 0.91836$; $X_2 = 0.081636$

The final result is $X_2 = 0.08164$ or 0.082

Molal solubility:

$$m = \frac{1000 X_2}{M_1 (1 - X_2)} = \frac{1000 \times 0.08164}{88.1 (1 - 0.08164)} = 1.01 \; molal$$

The activity is equal to the ideal solubility, $a_2 = X_2^i = 0.1802$

The activity coefficient is $\gamma_2 = \frac{a_2}{X_2} = \frac{0.1802}{0.08164} = 2.21$

PROBLEM 10.18. For acetone, the activity coefficient is

$$\gamma_2 = \frac{X_2^i}{X_2} = \frac{0.444}{0.378} = 1.2$$

Analogous calculations give the activity coefficients in the other solvents. The results are shown in Table P10 – 5. Naphthalene forms an ideal solution in chlorobenzene, since γ is equal to unity. In the other solvents the solubility is smaller than the ideal value, γ being larger than unity.

PROBLEM 10.19. (a) Pascal (Pa) $= N\,m^{-2} = J\,m^{-1}\,m^{-2} = J\,m^{-3}$

$$1 \; cal = 4.184 \; J; \quad 1\left(\frac{cal}{cm^3}\right) = 4.184 \times 10^6 \; J\,m^{-3} = 4.184 \times 10^6 \; Pa = 4.184 \; MPa;$$

$$1 \left(\frac{cal}{cm^3}\right)^{\frac{1}{2}} = (4.184 \ MPa)^{\frac{1}{2}} = 2.0455 \ (MPa)^{\frac{1}{2}}$$

The conversion factor is $\left(\frac{cal}{cm^3}\right)^{\frac{1}{2}} = 2.0455 \ (MPa)^{\frac{1}{2}}$

(b) Chloroform, 9.3 $(cal/cm^3)^{1/2}$ x $\dfrac{2.0455 \times (MPa)^{1/2}}{(cal/cm^3)^{1/2}} = 19.0 \ (MPa)^{1/2}$

Caffeine, 14.1 $(cal/cm^3)^{1/2}$ x $\dfrac{2.0455 \times (MPa)^{1/2}}{(cal/cm^3)^{1/2}} = 28.8 \ (MPa)^{1/2}$

Tolbutamide, 10.9 $(cal/cm^3)^{1/2}$ x $\dfrac{2.0455 \times (MPa)^{1/2}}{(cal/cm^3)^{1/2}} = 22.3 \ (MPa)^{1/2}$

Hydrocortisone, 12.4 $(cal/cm^3)^{1/2}$ x $\dfrac{2.0455 \times (MPa)^{1/2}}{(cal/cm^3)^{1/2}} = 25.4 \ (MPa)^{1/2}$

PROBLEM 10.20. (a)

$$V_2 = 104.3 \ \frac{cm^3}{mole} \times \frac{10^{-6} m^3}{cm^3} = 104.3 \times 10^{-6} \ \frac{m^3}{mole}$$

$$\Delta H_f = 4302 \ \frac{cal}{mole} \times 4.184 \ \frac{J}{cal} = 17999.6 \ J/mole = 18,000 \ J/mole$$

$$V_1 = 18.015 \ cm^3/mole \times (10^{-6} \ m^3)/cm^3 = 18.015 \times 10^{-6} \ m^3/mole$$

$$\delta_1 = 23.4 \ (cal/cm^3)^{1/2} \times \frac{2.0455 \times (MPa)^{1/2}}{(cal/cm)^{1/2}} = 47.9 \ (MPa)^{1/2}$$

$$\delta_2 = 11.5 \ (cal/cm^3)^{1/2} \times \frac{2.0455 \times (MPa)^{1/2}}{(cal/cm)^{1/2}} = 23.5 \ (MPa)^{1/2}$$

(b) The ideal solubility is:

$$\ln X_2^i = \frac{-17999.6 \ J \ mole^{-1}}{8.3143 \ J \ ^{\circ}K^{-1} mole^{-1}} \left(\frac{395.6 - 298.15}{395.6 \times 298.15}\right) = -1.7887$$

Using the Hildebrand equation and the SI units obtained in part **(a)**:

$$-\ln X_2 = 1.7887 + \frac{104.3 \times 10^{-6} \ (m^3/mole) \ (1)^2}{8.3143 \ J ^{\circ}K^{-1} mole^{-1} \times 298.15 ^{\circ}K} (47.9 - 23.5)^2$$

$$= 5.7968; \ X_2 = 0.00304$$

$$\text{molality} = \frac{1000 \ X_2}{M_1 \ (1 - X_2)} = \frac{1000 \times 0.00304}{18.015 \ (1 - 0.00304)} = 0.169 \ \text{mole/kg water}$$

PROBLEM 10.21. The internal pressure, P_i is

$$P_i = \left(\frac{\Delta H_v - RT}{V}\right) = \left(\frac{6682 - 592.4837}{60.4}\right) \cong 101 \ (cal/cm^3)$$

The solubility paramater is $\delta = (P_i)^{1/2} = 10 \ (cal/cm^3)^{1/2}$

PROBLEM 10.22. n–Hexane:

$a = 24.39 \ liter^2 \ atm \ mole^{-2}$; the molar volume is $131.6 \ cm^3 \ mole^{-1}$.

$(24.39 \ liter^2 \ atm \ mole^{-2}) \times (24.2179 \ cal/liter \ atm)$

$= 590.67 \ cal \ liter \ mole^{-2} = 590.67 \times 10^3 \ cal \ cm^3 \ mole^{-2}$;

$$\delta = \left(\frac{a}{V^2}\right)^{\frac{1}{2}} = \left(\frac{590.67 \times 10^3 \ cal \ cm^3 \ mole^{-2}}{(131.6)^2 \ (cm^3 mole^{-1})^2}\right)^{\frac{1}{2}} = 5.8 \ (cal/cm^3)^{1/2}$$

Benzene:

$a = 18.00 \ liter^2 \ atm \ mole^{-2}$; the molar volume is $89.4 \ cm^3 \ mole^{-1}$.

$(18.0 \ liter^2 \ atm \ mole^{-1}) \times (24.2179 \ cal/liter \ atm)$

$= 435.9 \ cal \ liter \ mole^{-2} = 435.9 \times 10^3 \ cal \ cm^3 \ mole^{-2}$; $\delta^2 = (a/V^2)$ and

$$\delta = \left(\frac{a}{V^2}\right)^{\frac{1}{2}} = \left(\frac{435.9 \times 10^3 \ cal \ cm^3 \ mole^{-2}}{(89.40)^2 \ (cm^3 mole^{-1})^2}\right)^{\frac{1}{2}} = 7.4 \ (cal/cm^3)^{1/2}$$

This method underestimates the value of δ

PROBLEM 10.23. Using equation (10–44),

$W_{(calc)} = 79.411400 + 1.868572(12.70) + 0.435648(12.70)^2 = 173.40793$

and $-\log X_2 = 1.1646 + 0.09467[12.70^2 + 13.8^2 - (2 \times 173.40793)]$

$= 1.62982$; $X_2 = 0.0235$

About 7 significant figures are required in the terms of the regression equations to calculate the solubilities using the Hildebrand technique. The answer may then be rounded to three significant figures.

PROBLEM 10.24. (a) Using equation (10–44),

$W_{(calc)} = 79.411400 + 1.868572(17.07) + 0.435648(17.07)^2 = 238.24917$

Using equation (10–45):

$W_{(calc)} = 15.075279 + 17.627903(17.07) - 0.966827(17.07)^2 + 0.053912(17.07)^3$

$- 0.000758(17.07)^4 = 238.06175$

(b)　Using $W_{(calc)}$ obtained from the quadratic equation,

$-\log X_2 = 1.1646 + 0.093711[17.07^2 + 13.8^2 - (2 \times 238.24917)] = 1.66376$

$X_2 = 0.02169$

$$M = \frac{1000\,\rho\,X_2}{M_1\,(1 - X_2) + X_2 M_2} = \frac{1000 \times 1.0439 \times 0.02169}{51.3\,(1 - 0.02169) + (0.02169)\,(194.19)}$$

M = 0.42 mole/liter.

Using $W_{(calc)}$ obtained from the quartic equation,

$-\log X_2 = 1.1646 + 0.093711[17.07^2 + 13.8^2 - (2 \times 238.06175)] = 1.69889$

$X_2 = 0.0200$

$$M = \frac{1000 \times 1.0493 \times 0.0200}{51.3\,(1 - 0.0200) + (0.0200)\,(194.19)} = 0.387\ mole/\ell$$

PROBLEM 10.25.　For ketoprofen in the chloroform-ethanol mixture, 70:30,

$$A = \frac{V_2 \phi_1^2}{2.303\,RT} = \frac{196\ cm^3 mole^{-1} \times (0.6694)^2}{2.303 \times 1.9872 \times 298.15} = 0.0644$$

$$\frac{-\log (X_2^i / X_2)}{A} = \delta_1{}^2 + \delta_2{}^2 - 2\,W$$

$-1.3354 = (10.32)^2 + (9.8)^2 - 2W; \qquad W = 101.9389$

$\delta_1 \delta_2 = 101.136; \qquad \dfrac{W}{\delta_1 \delta_2} = 1.0079$

For the chloroform-ethanol mixture, 50:50,

$A = 0.0668, \qquad W = 108.7395, \qquad \delta_1 \delta_2 = 107.800; \qquad \dfrac{W}{\delta_1 \delta_2} = 1.0087.$

PROBLEM 10.26.　Sulfamethoxypyridazine in benzene,

$$A = \frac{V_2 \phi_1^2}{2.303\,RT} = \frac{172.5\ cm^3 mole^{-1} \times (0.9999)^2}{2.303 \times 1.9872 \times 298.15} = 0.1264$$

$$\frac{-\log (X_2^i / X_2)}{A} = \delta_1{}^2 + \delta_2{}^2 - 2\,W$$

$17.0692 = (9.07)^2 + (12.89)^2 - 2W; \qquad W = 115.6739$

$\delta_1 \delta_2 = 116.9123; \qquad \dfrac{W}{\delta_1 \delta_2} = 0.9894$

<u>In benzyl alcohol,</u>

$A = 0.1204$, $W = 151.6831$, $\delta_1\delta_2 = 150.0396$; $\dfrac{W}{\delta_1\delta_2} = 1.0110$.

Notice that W is less than $\delta_1\delta_2$ in benzene and that W is larger than $\delta_1\delta_2$ in benzyl alcohol. The solubility in benzene is therefore less than the ideal solubility.

PROBLEM 10.27. (a)   Figure P10-3 shows a plot of the molar solubility, S, at 20°C and 37°C. As observed in the Figure, both sets of data follow a linear relationship. Therefore, using least squares, at 20°C,

$S_1 = 0.013 - 1.3 \times 10^{-4}$ (% glucose)
$(r^2 = 1.000)$

At 37°C,

$S_2 = 0.022 - 1.8 \times 10^{-4}$(% glucose)
$(r^2 = 0.998)$

where S_1 and S_2 are the molar solubilities at 20°C and 37°C, respectively.

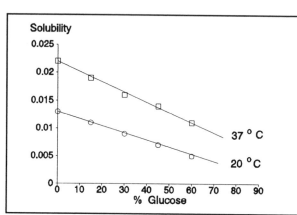

Figure P10-3 for Problem 10.27

As expected, the intercepts are equal to the solubility in water at 20°C and 37°C, respectively, as shown in the table found with problem 10.27.

Glucose decreases the solubility of sorbic acid (negative slope) as its concentration increases. The effect is slightly more pronounced at higher temperature (the slope at 37°C is steeper).

(b)   The free energy change in a saturated solution in water is

$\Delta G^{\circ}_{w} = -RT \ln X_w$, or in molarity,

$\Delta G^{\circ}_{w} = -RT \ln S_w$

and in the glucose solution

$\Delta G^{\circ}_{s} = -RT \ln S_s$

Where w stands for water and s for the glucose solution.

Therefore, the free energy change from water to the glucose solution, i. e. the free energy of transfer is

$$\Delta G^{\circ}_{tr} = \Delta G^{\circ}_{s} - \Delta G^{\circ}_{w} = -RT (\ln S_s - \ln S_w) = -RT \ln \frac{S_s}{S_w}$$

The enthalpy change, according to the van't Hoff expression at two temperatures for water is:

$$\ln \frac{S_{w_2}}{S_{w_1}} = \frac{\Delta H_w^o}{R}\left(\frac{T_2 - T_1}{T_2 T_1}\right)$$

and for the glucose solution,

$$\ln \frac{S_{s_2}}{S_{s_1}} = \frac{\Delta H_s^o}{R}\left(\frac{T_2 - T_1}{T_2 T_1}\right)$$

The enthalpy change of transfer from water to the glucose solution is:

$$\Delta H_{tr}^o = \Delta H_s^o - \Delta H_w^o = \frac{R\ln\left(S_{s_2}/S_{s_1}\right)}{\left(\dfrac{T_2 - T_1}{T_2 T_1}\right)} - \frac{R\ln\left(S_{w_2}/S_{w_1}\right)}{\left(\dfrac{T_2 - T_1}{T_2 T_1}\right)} =$$

$$\frac{R}{\left(\dfrac{T_2 - T_1}{T_2 T_1}\right)}\ln\left(\frac{\left(S_{s_2}/S_{s_1}\right)}{\left(S_{w_2}/S_{w_1}\right)}\right) \quad or \quad \ln\frac{\left(S_{s_2}/S_{s_1}\right)}{\left(S_{w_2}/S_{w_1}\right)} = \frac{\Delta H_{tr}^o}{R}\left(\frac{T_2 - T_1}{T_1 T_2}\right)$$

(c)   At 20°C, $\Delta G_{tr}^o = -1.9872(20 + 273.15)\ln\dfrac{0.007}{0.013} = +360.6$ cal/mole

At 37°C, $\Delta G_{tr}^o = -1.9872(37 + 273.15)\ln\dfrac{0.014}{0.022} = +278.6$ cal/mole

The enthalpy change of tranfer is

$$\ln\frac{\left(\dfrac{0.014}{0.022}\right)}{\left(\dfrac{0.007}{0.013}\right)} = \frac{\Delta H_{tr}^o}{1.9872}\left(\frac{310.15 - 293.15}{310.15 \times 293.15}\right); \quad \text{solving for } \Delta H^o{}_{tr} \text{ we obtain}$$

$\Delta H^o{}_{tr} = 1775$ cal/mole

$\Delta G^o{}_{tr}$ and $\Delta H^o{}_{tr}$ are both positive, indicating that the process is not spontaneous in the standard state. The dissolution process of sorbic acid is unfavorable with addition of glucose, a result which is corroborated by the decrease of solubility as the concentration of glucose increases.

PROBLEM 10.28. (a) $T = 193°K$ and $T_f = (-56) + 273 = 217°K$

$$\ln X_2{}^i = -\frac{\Delta H_f}{R}\left(\frac{T_f - T}{T_f T}\right) = -\frac{1900}{1.9872}\left(\frac{217 - 193}{217 \times 193}\right) = -0.5479$$

$X_2{}^i = 0.5782$

(b) The equation relating the density, ρ and the temperature (°C) is

$\rho = 0.80628 - 8.42707 \times 10^{-4}t$

The density of ethanol at $-80°C$ is calculated from the equation,

$\rho = 0.80628 (-8.42707 \times 10^{-4})(-80) = 0.87370$

The molar volume, V_1, at $-80°C$ is $V_1 = \dfrac{46.07 \ g/mole}{0.87370 \ g/cm^3} = 52.73 \ cm^3/mole$

(c) The solubility parameter of ethanol at $-80°C$ is:

$\delta_{-80°} = 12.8\left(\dfrac{0.78521}{0.87370}\right)^{1.25} = 11.2 \ (cal/cm^3)^{\frac{1}{2}}$

The solubility parameter for CO_2 is:

$\delta_{CO_2} = \left(\dfrac{\Delta H_v - RT}{V}\right)^{\frac{1}{2}} = \left(\dfrac{3460 - (1.9872 \times 193)}{38}\right)^{\frac{1}{2}} = 9.0$

(d) The solubility of CO_2 at $-80°C$ is calculated from the Hildebrand equation, assuming that $\phi_1 = 1$ in the first approximation,

$-\ln X_2 = 0.5479 + \dfrac{38 (1)^2}{1.9872 \times 193} (11.2 - 9.0)^2 = 1.02745$

$X_2 = 0.35792$; for the second approximation,

$\phi_1 = \dfrac{(1 - X_2) 52.73}{(1 - X_2) 52.73 + (X_2 \times 38)} = \dfrac{0.64208 \times 52.73}{0.64208 \times 52.73 + (0.35792 \times 38)}$

$= 0.71341$. Then, we use the calculated $\phi_1 = 0.71341$ to compute X_2 from the Hildebrand equation; since all the parameters are constant except ϕ_1 the Hildebrand equation reduces to:
$-\ln X_2 = 0.5479 + 0.47955(\phi_1)^2$:
$-\ln X_2 = 0.5479 + 0.47955(0.71341)^2 = 0.79197 \ ; \ X_2 = 0.45295$

Following these steps, and after eight iterations (using a hand calculator), one obtains $X_2 = 0.4887$ (mole fraction), the solubility of CO_2 in ethanol at $-80°C$.

(e) The result, expressed in molality is

$m = \dfrac{1000 X_2}{M_1 (1 - X_2)} = \dfrac{1000 \times 0.4887}{46.07 (1 - 0.4887)} = 20.7 \ \dfrac{moles \ CO_2}{kg \ ethanol}$

PROBLEM 10.29. Using equation (10 – 46),

$\ln c_1 - \ln c_2 = \dfrac{1}{v}\left\{\dfrac{\Delta H_{soln}}{R}\left(\dfrac{T_1 - T_2}{T_1 T_2}\right)\right\}$

$\ln (21.52) - \ln c_2 = \dfrac{1}{3}\left\{\dfrac{13500}{1.9872}\left(\dfrac{273.15 - 298.15}{273.15 \times 298.15}\right)\right\}$

$3.06898 - \ln c_2 = -0.69514; \ \ln c_2 = 3.76412$

Table P10−6 for Problem 10.30.

$\ln m_2$	−2.3289	−1.9331	−1.4828
$1/T$ (°K^{-1}) x 10^3	3.661	3.532	3.411

c_2 = exp(3.76412) = 43.13 g/(100 g water) = 43.13 g/(hectogram water).
(Note: 1 hectogram = 1 hg = 100 gram).

PROBLEM 10.30. (a)   The data needed for the regression analysis are shown in Table P10−6. The regression equation is:

$\ln m_2$ = 10.0355 − 3380.9 $\dfrac{1}{T}$, r^2 = 0.9969

ΔH_{soln} = (−slope) x R = (3380.9)(1.9872) = 6719 cal/mole

At 30°C (303.15 °K), $\dfrac{1}{T}$ = 3.299 x 10^{-3},

$\ln m_2$ = 10.0355 − (3380.9)(3.299 x 10^{-3}) = −1.1181
m_2 = exp(−1.1181) = 0.3269 ≈ 0.327 molal. The experimental value is 0.326 molal.

PROBLEM 10.31.

$$Ag_2CrO_4 \rightleftharpoons 2\ Ag^+ + CrO_4^=$$
$$x \qquad 2x \qquad x$$

K_{sp} = (2x)^{2}x;   2 x 10^{-12} = 4x^3
x^3 = 0.5 x 10^{-12};   x = 7.9 x 10^{-5}

PROBLEM 10.32. (a)

$Mg(OH)_2 \rightleftharpoons 2\ OH^- + Mg^{++}$
K_{sp} = [Mg][OH$^-$]^2;   1.4 x 10^{-11} = (2x)^2(x)

$x = \sqrt[3]{\dfrac{1.4 \times 10^{-11}}{4}}$ = 1.5 x 10^{-4} mole/liter

(b)   1.5 x 10^{-4} mole/liter x 58.34 g/mole = 8.8 x 10^{-3} g/liter;
8.8 x 10^{-3} g/liter = 8.8 x 10^{-4} g/deciliter.
(Note 1 deciliter = 10^{-1} liter = 100 ml).

PROBLEM 10.33. (a)   Brequinar sodium $\rightleftharpoons$ [Brequinar$^-$] + [Na$^+$]
K'_{sp} = (x)(x); 0.0751 = x^2.

Solubility, $x = \sqrt{0.0751} = 0.274$ mole/liter

(b) For a univalent electrolyte, μ = molar concentration = 0.274;

$$\log \gamma_{\pm} = -\frac{0.51\sqrt{0.274}}{1 + \sqrt{0.274}} = -0.175 ; \quad \gamma_{\pm} = 0.668$$

$K_{sp} = [\text{Brequinar}^-][\text{Na}^+](0.668)^2 = (0.274)(0.274)(0.668)^2 = 0.0335$

(c) The ionic strength with the addition of 0.05 M KCl is $0.274 + 0.05 = 0.324$,

$$\log \gamma_{\pm} = -\frac{0.51\sqrt{0.324}}{1 + \sqrt{0.324}} = -0.185 ; \quad \gamma_{\pm} = 0.653$$

Solubility $= \frac{\sqrt{K_{sp}}}{\gamma_{\pm}} = \frac{\sqrt{0.0335}}{0.653} = 0.280$ mole/liter

Note that KCl, a salt, having no ion common with brequinar sodium, increases the solubility because the activity coefficient is lowered.

PROBLEM 10.34. (a) $\Delta H_{soln} = \Delta H_{sublimation} + \Delta H_{hydration}$
$\Delta H_{soln} = 207 - 192 = 15$ kcal/mole for silver chloride.
Converting to kJ/mole,
$\Delta H_{soln} = 15$ kcal/mole x 4.184 kJ/kcal = 62.8 kJ/mole.
(b) Using equation (10-46),

$$\ln c_{25^\circ} - \ln c_{10^\circ} = \frac{1}{\nu}\left\{\frac{\Delta H_{soln}}{R}\left(\frac{T_{25^\circ} - T_{10^\circ}}{T_{10^\circ} T_{25^\circ}}\right)\right\}$$

$$\ln c_{25^\circ} - \ln(8.9 \times 10^{-5}) = \frac{1}{2}\left\{\frac{15000}{1.9872}\left(\frac{298.15 - 283.15}{298.15 \times 283.15}\right)\right\};$$

$\ln c_{25^\circ} = 0.6706 + \ln(8.9 \times 10^{-5}) = -8.65627;$
$c_{25^\circ} = 1.74 \times 10^{-4}$ g/deciliter.

PROBLEM 10.35. For KBr, $\Delta H_{soln} = 673 - 651 = 22$ kJ/mole
1 cal = 4.184 J; and 1 kcal = 4.184 kJ

$22 \text{ kJ} \frac{1 \ kcal}{4.184 \ (kJ/kcal)} = 5.3$ kcal/mole

For KCl, $\Delta H_{soln} = 699 - 686 = 13$ kJ/mole

$13 \text{ kJ} \frac{1 \ kcal}{4.184 \ (kJ/kcal)} = 3.1$ kcal/mole

PROBLEM 10.36. $BaSO_4 \rightleftarrows Ba^{++} + SO_4^{=}$

Solubility $= \dfrac{\sqrt{K_{sp}}}{\gamma_\pm} = \dfrac{\sqrt{1 \times 10^{-10}}}{0.23} = 4.3 \times 10^{-5}$ mole/liter

PROBLEM 10.37.

$\ln c_{50°} - \ln(2.08) = \left\{ \dfrac{3470}{1.9872} \left(\dfrac{323.15 - 308.15}{323.15 \times 308.15} \right) \right\};$

$\ln c_{50°} = 0.2630 + \ln(2.08) = 0.9954; \quad c_{50°} = 2.71$ molal

PROBLEM 10.38.

$pH_p = pK_a + \log \dfrac{S - S_o}{S_o} \; ; \quad S = \dfrac{50 \text{ g/}\ell}{304 \text{ g/mole}} = 0.164 \text{ M}$

$pH_p = 7.12 + \log \dfrac{0.164 - 0.002}{0.002} = 9.03$

PROBLEM 10.39.

$S = \dfrac{20 \text{ g/}\ell}{254.22 \text{ g/mole}} = 0.0787 \text{ M}; \quad S_o = \dfrac{2.2 \text{ g/}\ell}{232.23 \text{ g/mole}} = 0.009 \text{ M}$

$pH_p = pK_a + \log \dfrac{S - S_o}{S_o} = 7.6 + \log \dfrac{0.0787 - 0.009}{0.009} = 8.5$

PROBLEM 10.40.   (5 g/liter)/(339.8 g/mole) = 0.0147 M

$pH_p = pK_w - pK_b + \log \dfrac{S_o}{S - S_o} = 14 - 5.59 + \log \dfrac{0.0056}{0.0147 - 0.0056};$

$pH_p = 8.41 + \log(0.6154) = 8.20$

PROBLEM 10.41. (a)   The pK_a values of phenobarbital and its solubility at the several concentrations of alcohol are read from Figures 10 − 8 and 10 − 7, respectively. These values are listed in Table P10 − 7.

The molar concentration of sodium phenobarbital, S, is $\dfrac{30 \text{ g}}{254.22 \text{ g/mole}} = 0.118$ M.

At 10 % alcohol, the solubility of free phenobarbital is 0.19 g/(100 ml), and the molar solubility, S_o, is $\dfrac{1.9 \text{ g/}\ell}{232.23 \text{ g/mole}} = 0.008$ mole/liter. The pK_a value is 7.6 (Table P10 − 7).

The pH$_p$ is:

$$pH_p = pK_a + \log \frac{S - S_o}{S_o}$$

$$= 7.6 + \log \frac{0.118 - 0.008}{0.008} = 8.73$$

At 20 % alcohol, the solubility of phenobarbital is 0.29 g/(100 ml), as read from Figure 10−7; the molar solubility S$_o$ is

$$\frac{2.9 \ g/\ell}{232.23 \ g/mole} = 0.0125 \ \text{mole/liter}.$$

Using this value together with pK$_a$ at 20 % alcohol, pK$_a$ = 7.7 (Table P10−7), one obtains

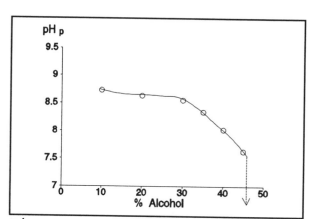

Figure P10-4 for Problem 10.41

$$pH_p = 7.7 + \log \frac{0.118 - 0.0125}{0.0125} = 8.63.$$

Table P10−7 gives the calculated values for pH$_p$, the minimum pH required for complete solubility of sodium phenobarbital at several concentrations of alcohol.

(b) The results are plotted in Figure P10−4. Note in the Figure that at 45 % to 50 % alcohol, the pH$_p$ tends to decrease sharply towards zero.

Table P10−7 for Problem 10.41.

% Alcohol	10	20	30	35	40	45	50
pK$_a$[a]	7.6	7.7	7.9	8	8.1	8.25	8.5
S (g/(100 ml)[b]	0.19	0.29	0.5	0.236	1.5	2.2	3.2
S$_o$ (mole/liter)	0.008	0.0125	0.0215	0.0370	0.0646	0.0947	0.138
pH$_p$	8.73	8.63	8.55	8.34	8.02	7.63	c

[a] Read from Figure 10-8.

[b] Read from Figure 10-7.

[c] These results show that at about 50 % alcohol and above, phenobarbital will not precipitate regardless of how low the pH.

PROBLEM 10.42. The molar concentration of codeine phosphate is

60 mg/5 ml = 12 g/liter; $\dfrac{12\ g/\ell}{406.37\ g/mole}$ = 0.0295 M of phosphate salt.

$$pH = pK_w - pK_b + \log\frac{S_o}{S - S_o} = 8.21 + \log\frac{0.0279}{0.0295 - 0.0279} = 9.45$$

The pH above which the free base precipitates from solution is 9.45.

PROBLEM 10.43. By alligation[a]:

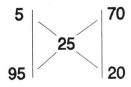

25 − 5 = 20 parts of 95 %

95 − 25 = 70 parts of 5 %. Then 70 parts + 20 parts = 90 parts.

$\dfrac{20\ parts}{90\ parts} = \dfrac{x}{60\ ml}$;   x = $\dfrac{20}{90}$×60 = 13.3 ml of USP alcohol.

$\dfrac{70\ parts}{90\ parts} = \dfrac{x}{60\ ml}$;   X = $\dfrac{70}{90}$×60 = 46.7 ml of 5 % alcohol.

PROBLEM 10.44.

$[H_3O^+]$ = $\sqrt{K_1 C}$ = $\sqrt{(4.0\times10^{-7})(1.0\times10^{-5})}$ = 2×10^{-6}; $pH = 5.7$

PROBLEM 10.45. (a)   pH = 5.12, $[H_3O^+]$ = 7.586 x 10^{-6};
K_a = 7.6 x 10^{-6}

The total solubility in the absence of surfactant is calculated from equation (10 − 73):

$$D_T^* = 0.15\left[\frac{7.6\times10^{-6} + 7.568\times10^{-6}}{7.586\times10^{-6}}\right] = 0.30\ g/\ell$$

(b) From equation (10 − 74), total solubility of drug in the presence of 3 % Tween 80 is

$$D_T = 0.30\left\{1 + 0.03\left[\frac{(7.6\times10^{-6})(15) + (7.586\times10^{-6})(79)}{7.586\times10^{-6} + 7.6\times10^{-6}}\right]\right\};$$

where K' and K'' are 79 and 19, respectively. The volume fraction of tween 80 is 0.03.

---

[a] Alligation is explained in W. Lowenthal, Metrology and Calculations, Chapter 9 in <u>Remington's Pharmaceutical Siences</u>, A. R. Gennaro, Editor, Mack, Easton, Pa, 1985, pp. 99, 100.

D_T = 0.723 g/liter. The presence of surfactant has increased the solubility 2.4 times.

(c) The fraction of sulfisoxazole solubilized in the Tween 80 micelles is

$$\frac{0.723 \ g/\ell - 0.30 \ g/\ell}{0.723 \ g/\ell} = 0.585$$

PROBLEM 10.46. (a) Using equation (10 – 101):

ΔS_f = 13.5 + 2.5(n – 5) = 13.5 + 2.5(6 – 5) = 16 e.u.

The partition coefficient of butyl p–hydroxybenzoate is

log K = 1.87 + (4 x 0.50) + (– 1.16) = 2.71

Using the Yalkowsky equation,

$$\log S = -\log K - 1.11 \frac{\Delta S_f (mp - 25)}{1364} + 0.54 =$$

$$-2.71 - 1.11 \frac{16 \ (68° - 25°)}{1364} + 0.54 = -2.7299; \quad S = 1.86 \times 10^{-3}$$

PROBLEM 10.47. For phenytoin, n = 6, and ΔS_f is:

ΔS_f = 13.5 + 2.5(n – 5) = 13.5 + 2.5(6 – 5) = 16 e.u

$$\alpha = 1 + \frac{10^{-8.30}}{10^{-7.1}} = 1 + \frac{5.01 \times 10^{-9}}{7.94 \times 10^{-8}} = 1.063$$

$$\log S = \frac{-16 \ (570.05° - 298.15°)}{2.303 \times 1.9872 \times 298.15} - \log(208.9) + \log(1.063) + 0.8$$

$$= -4.6835; \quad S = 2.07 \times 10^{-5}$$

(b) $\alpha = 1 + \dfrac{10^{-8.07}}{10^{-8.0}} = 1.85$

$$-1.956 = \frac{-12.67 \ (401.65° - 306.15°)}{2.303 \times 1.9872 \times 306.15} - \log K + \log (1.85) + 0.8$$

$$-1.956 = -0.8636 - \log K + 0.267 + 0.8 ; \quad \log K = 2.16, \text{ and } K = 144.5.$$

PROBLEM 10.48. $K = \dfrac{C_{et}}{C_{H_2O}} = 0.125 = \dfrac{[(0.15 - x)/100]}{(x/10)}$

where x is the amount of succinic acid in the aqueous phase.

1.25 x = 0.15 – x;   x = 0.0666 g in the aqueous phase

0.15 – 0.0666 = 0.083 g after first extraction.

For the second extraction, $0.125 = \dfrac{[(0.0833 - x)/100]}{(x/10)}$

2.25 x = 0.0833; x = 0.03703 g in the aqueous phase

0.0833 − 0.03703 = 0.046 in the ether layer after the second extraction.

PROBLEM 10.49. Using equation (10 − 105),

$$[HA_w] = \frac{C}{(K \times q) + 1 + \dfrac{K_a}{[H_3O^+]}} = \frac{500}{5.33 + 1 + \dfrac{6.3 \times 10^{-5}}{1 \times 10^{-5}}} ;$$

where the initial concentration, C is 500 mg/(100 ml) and $[H_3O^+]$ is 1 x 10^{-5} ; K x q = 5.33 since q = V_o/V_w = 1 (50 % oil − in − water emulsion).

$[HA]_w$ = 39.58828 mg/100 ml or 0.396 mg/ml.

PROBLEM 10.50. $C = \left[K''^2 q [HA]_w + 1 + \dfrac{K_a}{[H_3O^+]} \right] [HA]_w =$

$$\left[(15)^2 (0.25) \frac{0.65\ g}{74.08\ g/mole} + 1 + \frac{1.34 \times 10^{-5}}{3.16 \times 10^{-4}} \right] \frac{0.65}{74.08} = 0.0135\ M$$

In grams per ml $= \dfrac{0.0135 \times 74.08}{1000} = 1 \times 10^{-3}$ g/ml = 1.0 mg/ml.

PROBLEM 10.51. **(a)** The data needed are presented Table P10 − 8 and plotted in Figure P10 − 5.

Using linear regression, at 27°, $\dfrac{1}{K_{obs}} = 0.75515 + 6.028 \times 10^6 [H_3O^+]$; r^2 = 0.999

intercept $= \dfrac{1}{K_{in}}$; $K_{in} = \dfrac{1}{0.75515}$ = 1.324

slope $= \dfrac{1}{K_{in} K_a}$; $K_a = \dfrac{1}{1.324 \times 6.028 \times 10^6}$ = 1.25 x 10^{-7} ; pK_a = 6.90

At 30°, $\dfrac{1}{K_{obs}} = 0.69759 + 4.534 \times 10^6 [H_3O^+]$; r^2 = 0.998

intercept $= \dfrac{1}{K_{in}}$; $K_{in} = \dfrac{1}{0.69759}$ = 1.433

slope $= \dfrac{1}{K_{in} K_a}$; $K_a = \dfrac{1}{1.433 \times 4.534 \times 10^6}$ = 1.54 x 10^{-7} ; pK_a = 6.81

At 40°, $\dfrac{1}{K_{obs}} = 0.47463 + 3.3540 \times 10^6 [H_3O^+]$; r^2 = 0.9996

Table P10−8 for Problem 10.51

$[H_3O^+]$ (x 10^7)	5.62	3.16	2.00	1.41	1.00	0.56
t (°C)			$1/K_{obs}$			
27	4.17	2.63	1.92	1.59	1.39	1.12
30	3.23	2.17	1.61	1.28	1.19	0.94
40	–	1.54	1.14	0.94	0.81	0.67

Table P10−9 for Problem 10.51.

$\frac{1}{T}$ (x10^3)	3.332	3.229	3.193
ln K_{in}	0.2807	0.3598	0.7448

intercept $= \dfrac{1}{K_{in}};$ $K_{in} = \dfrac{1}{0.47463} = 2.106$

slope $= \dfrac{1}{K_{in}K_a};$ $K_a = \dfrac{1}{2.106 \times 3.3540 \times 10^6} = 1.42 \times 10^{-7};$ $pK_a = 6.85$

(b) The data needed are shown in Table P10−9.

The equation is: ln $K_{in} = 11.6302 - 3410.5 \dfrac{1}{T}$

slope $= -3410.5 = -\dfrac{\Delta H°}{R};$

$\Delta H° = 6777$ cal/mole $= 6.8$ kcal/mole

intercept $= 11.6302 = \dfrac{\Delta S°}{R};$

$\Delta S° = (1.9872)(11.6302) = 23$ cal/(mole deg)
The standard free energy is calculated from
$\Delta G° = \Delta H° - T \Delta S°.$

At 27°,

$\Delta G° = 6777.4 - (300.15 \times 23.11)$

$= -159$ cal/mole.

The results at the other two temperatures are:

At 30°, $\Delta G° = -228$ cal/mole

At 40°, $\Delta G° = -460$ cal/mole.

$\Delta H°$ is positive which mitigates against the partitioning process, yet $\Delta S°$ is sufficiently positive to provide a spontaneous reaction. The negative $\Delta G°$ values corroborate this conclusion that the process is spontaneous (for the solute in its standard state).

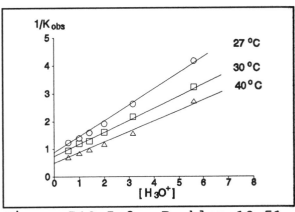

Figure P10-5 for Problem 10.51

The large positive $\Delta S°$ value suggests that pilocarpine base is solvated in the aqueous phase in an orderly structure, which is broken down to a more random arrangement of drug and solvent in the octanol phase. A suggested reason for the large positive $\Delta H°$ is the following. Removal of the pilocarpine molecules from the surrounding water molecules to which they are hydrogen bonded in the aqueous phase (a process of desolvation), requires a considerable absorption of energy, represented by a positive $\Delta H°$. As the free pilocarpine molecules then pass into the octanol phase they are resolvated, together with a liberation of energy, i.e., a negative $\Delta H°$. But the drug is much more weakly bound in octanol than in the aqueous phase so that the overall process of desolvation of the solute in water and resolvation in octanol involves a large net absorption of energy, resulting in a large positive $\Delta H°$ value (see A. K. Mitra and T. J. Mikkelson, J. Pharm. Sci. **77**, 771, 1988).

Chapter 11
Complexation and Protein Binding

PROBLEM 11.1. From equations (11 − 14) and (11 − 15),

$p[A] = \log K_1$ at $\bar{n} = \frac{1}{2}$ and $p[A] = \log K_2$ at $\bar{n} = \frac{3}{2}$.

From Figure P11 − 1, at $\bar{n} = \frac{1}{2}$

$\log K_1 = 3.9$.

At $\bar{n} = \frac{3}{2}$, $\log K_2 = 2.97$.

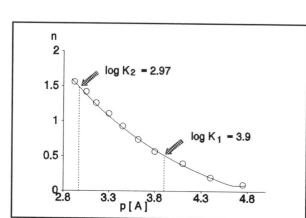

Figure P11-1 for Problem 11.1

The overall stability constant is

$\beta = K_1 K_2;$ $\log \beta = 3.9 + 2.97 = 6.87$

PROBLEM 11.2. $\log \dfrac{K_2}{K_1} = \dfrac{\Delta H^\circ}{2.303\ R}\left(\dfrac{T_2 - T_1}{T_2 T_1}\right)$

$9.79 - 9.27 = \dfrac{\Delta H^\circ}{2.303 \times 1.9872}\left(\dfrac{313.15 - 298.15}{313.15 \times 298.15}\right)$

$\Delta H^\circ = 14813$ cal/mole $= 14.8$ kcal/mole

$\Delta G^\circ = -2.303\ RT \log K = -(2.303)(1.9872)(313.15)(9.79)$

$= -14030$ cal/mole $= -14$ kcal/mole at 40°C.

$\Delta S^\circ = \dfrac{\Delta H^\circ - \Delta G^\circ}{T} = \dfrac{14813 - (-14030)}{313.15} = 92$ cal/(mole deg)

PROBLEM 11.3. Complexed benzoic acid = total benzoic − free benzoic
$= (20.4 \times 10^{-3}) - (11.94 \times 10^{-3}) = 8.46 \times 10^{-3}$ M.
Since we have a 1:1 complex, complexed benzoic = complexed caffeine;
[caffeine] = [total caffeine] − [complexed benzoic] =
$(2.69 \times 10^{-2}) - (8.46 \times 10^{-3}) = 1.84 \times 10^{-2}$ M

$K = \dfrac{8.46 \times 10^{-3}}{(11.94 \times 10^{-3})\ (1.84 \times 10^{-2})} = 38.5$

PROBLEM 11.4. Phenobarbital content of the complex = total phenobarbital added − phenobarbital dissolved at point B = $(21.5 \times 10^{-3}) - (6.5 \times 10^{-3}) = 15 \times 10^{-3}$ M.

Stoichiometric ratio = $\dfrac{PGE\ in\ complex}{Phenobarbital\ in\ complex} = \dfrac{30 \times 10^{-3}}{15 \times 10^{-3}} = \dfrac{2}{1}$ = 2:1 complex

PROBLEM 11.5. Sulfathiazole complexed = $(3.27 \times 10^{-3}) - (2.27 \times 10^{-3}) = 1.00 \times 10^{-3}$; since it is a 1:1 complex, complexed sulfathiazole must equal complexed caffeine. Free caffeine = total caffeine − caffeine complexed
= $(3.944 \times 10^{-2}) - (1.00 \times 10^{-3}) = 3.84 \times 10^{-2}$ M

$K = \dfrac{1.00 \times 10^{-3}}{(2.27 \times 10^{-3})\ (3.84 \times 10^{-2})} = 11.5$

PROBLEM 11.6. Complexed butyl paraben = $(3.72 \times 10^{-3}) - (0.58 \times 10^{-3}) = 3.14 \times 10^{-3}$ M; since this is a 1:1 complex, complexed butyl paraben must equal complexed caffeine.

Free caffeine = total caffeine − complexed caffeine
= $(6.25 \times 10^{-2}) - (3.14 \times 10^{-3}) = 5.94 \times 10^{-2}$ M

$K = \dfrac{3.14 \times 10^{-3}}{(5.94 \times 10^{-2})\ (0.58 \times 10^{-3})} = 91.1$

PROBLEM 11.7. (a) The plot is shown in Figure P11 − 2.

(b) The solubility of the anthraquinone is given by the value of the intercept extrapolating the first linear part, AB, graphically. To get a better result, the intercept is calculated by regressing the concentration of 1,8 dihydroanthraquinone (y) versus the concentration of cyclodextrin (x).

Figure P11-2 for Problem 11.7

The equation obtained is:
$y = 1.67 \times 10^{-6} + 8.29 \times 10^{-4} x$
($r^2 = 0.949$). From the intercept, $S_o = 1.7 \times 10^{-6}$ M. The authors report a value of 1×10^{-6} M

(c) From the regression equation, the apparent stability constant is (see T. Higuchi and K. Connors, Adv. Anal. Chem. Instr., 4, 117, 1965):

$K = \dfrac{slope}{intercept\ (1 - slope)} = \dfrac{8.29 \times 10^{-4}}{(1.67 \times 10^{-6})\ (1 - 8.29 \times 10^{-4})} = 497$ M^{-1}

Table P11 – 1 for Problem 11.8.[a]

$[A_t] - [A_o]$ (x10^5)	$\log([A_t] - [A_o])$	$\log [D_t]$
1.382	– 4.860	– 0.787
3.242	– 4.489	– 0.333
6.827	– 4.166	– 0.106
19.966	– 3.700	0.193
76.645	– 3.116	0.494
206.2	– 2.686	0.672
434.2	– 2.362	0.800
858.0	– 2.067	0.895

PROBLEM 11.8. (a) The data needed for regression analysis are given in Table P11 – 1.

The regression of $\log([A_t] - [A_o])$ versus $\log [D_t]$ gives the results:

$\log([A_t] - [A_o]) = 1.695 \log [D_t] - 3.818$ ($r^2 = 0.966$)

Taking the log of equation (11 – 53),

$$\log([A_t] - [A_o]) = \frac{m}{2} \log [D_t] + \log K$$

Therefore, slope $= 1.695 = \dfrac{m}{2}$ and m $= 1.695 \times 2 = 3.390$. (Number of hexanoic acid molecules per griseofulvin molecule in the complex).

(b) From equations (11 – 53) and (11 – 54),

intercept $= -3.818 = \log K = \log K_m - \dfrac{m}{2} \log K_d - \dfrac{m}{2} \log 2$

Solving for $\log K_m$,

$$\log K_m = -3.818 + \left(\frac{3.390}{2} \log 6000\right) + \left(\frac{3.390}{2} \log 2\right) = 3.0962;$$

$K_m = $ antilog $(3.0962) = 1248 \, M^{-1}$

---

[a] If the work required to obtain the data in columns 2 and 3 of Table P11-1 seems excessive for the student, the instructor may ask the student to compute every other value (4 values in all), or he/she can present the student with Table P11-1 as a handout to help reduce the work.

PROBLEM 11.9. The regression equations are:

At 2°C : $\dfrac{A_o}{A} = 0.0123\ \dfrac{1}{D_o} + 0.0097$

At 18°C : $\dfrac{A_o}{A} = 0.0187\ \dfrac{1}{D_o} + 0.0097$

At 25°C : $\dfrac{A_o}{A} = 0.0216\ \dfrac{1}{D_o} + 0.0097$

At 37°C : $\dfrac{A_o}{A} = 0.0277\ \dfrac{1}{D_o} + 0.0097$

From the Benesi – Hildebrand equation, intercept $= \dfrac{1}{\epsilon}$, and slope $= \dfrac{1}{\epsilon\ K}$. The equations have a common intercept[a], 0.0097, $\epsilon = \dfrac{1}{0.0097} = 103.1$. The slope varies with temperature. At 2°C, slope $= 0.0123 = \dfrac{1}{(103.1)\ K}$; $K = 0.79$.

Analogous calculations for the other three temperatures give K = 0.54, 0.45 and 0.35 at 18°C, 25°C, and 37°C, respectively.

PROBLEM 11.10.

At 2°C, $\Delta G^\circ = -RT\ \ln K = -(1.9872)(275.15)(\ln 0.97) = +16.7$ cal/mole

At 18°C, $\Delta G^\circ = -(1.9872)(291.15)(-0.3147) = +182.1$ cal/mole

At 37°C, $\Delta G^\circ = -(1.9872)(310.15)(-0.5621) = +346.5$ cal/mole

ΔH° is calculated from a regression of ln K versus $\dfrac{1}{T}$. The data needed are presented in table: P11 – 2

Table P11 – 2 for Problem 11.10.

ln K	−0.0305	−0.3147	−0.5621
$\dfrac{1}{T}$ (x 10³)	3.634	3.435	3.224

---

[a] The authors report that ϵ is independent of temperature. However, due to experimental error, ϵ varies slightly, the value, 103.1 given in the paper being an average value. The data given in this problem are not the experimental values but rather they have been back-calculated from the constants in Table I given by the authors in their paper. For this reason we obtained exactly the same value for ϵ at the four different temperatures.

The equation is:

$$\ln K = 1295.3 \frac{1}{T} - 4.746; \quad slope = \frac{-\Delta H^\circ}{R}; \quad \Delta H^\circ = -(1295.3)(1.9872) = -2574$$

cal/mole. The intercept is $= \frac{\Delta S^\circ}{R}$; $\Delta S^\circ = (-4.746)(1.9872) = -9.4$ u.e.

ΔG° is small (see above) and positive although ΔH° is large and negative. This is because of the high negative entropy change, which indicates a change to a more ordered structure when the complex is formed. (See p. 984 in the paper, J. Pharm. Sci, <u>65</u>, 982, 1976).

PROBLEM 11.11. ΔH° is calculated from a regression of log K against 1/T. The data needed are presented in Table P11 – 3.

$$\log K = -\frac{\Delta H^\circ}{2.303\,R} \frac{1}{T} + constant; \quad the\ regression\ gives\ \log K = 861.51 \frac{1}{T} - 3.2365;$$

$$\Delta H^\circ = (-slope)(1.9872)(2.303) = (-861.51)(1.9872)(2.303) = -3943\ cal/mole.$$

At 2°C, $\Delta G^\circ = -(2.303)RT \log K$

$$= -(2.303)(1.9872)(275.15)(-0.1024) = 128.95\ cal/mole.$$

For the other temperatures, ΔG° is 378.43, 473.22, and 647.13 cal/mole at 18°C (291.15°K), 25°C (298.15 °K) and 37°C (310.15°K), respectively.

The entropy change at 2°C is

$$\Delta S^\circ = \frac{\Delta H^\circ - \Delta G^\circ}{T} = \frac{-3943 - 128.95}{275.15} = -14.80\ cal/mole\ deg.$$

For the other temperatures, analogous calculations give -14.84, -14.81 and -14.80 cal/(mole deg), at 18°C, 25°C and 37°C, respectively.

PROBLEM 11.12. (a) Assuming that ΔH° and ΔS° are constant over the temperature range, they can be computed from the slope and the intercept, respectively of a regression of ln K against $\frac{1}{T}$. (Table P11 – 4)

The equation thus obtained is

Table P11 – 3 for Problem 11.11.

log K	−0.1024	−0.2840	−0.3468	−0.4559
$1/T \times 10^3$	3.634	3.435	3.354	3.224

Table P11 − 4 for Problem 11.12.

ln K	1.2528	0.8329	0.3507
1/T (x 10^3)	3.595	3.470	3.354

ln K $= 3738.2 \frac{1}{T} - 12.1706$; $\Delta H^\circ = -(slope)(R) = (3738.2)(1.9872) = -7428.6$

cal/mole or − 7.4 kcal/mole.

$\Delta S^\circ = (intercept)(R) = (-12.1706)(1.9872) = -24.2$ cal/(mole deg)

At 5°C, $\Delta G^\circ = -RT \ln K = -(1.9872)(278.15)(1.2528)$

$= -692.5$ cal/mole $= -0.69$ kcal/mole

Analogous calculations using ln K values from Table P11 − 4, give ΔG° at 15°C and 25°C to be − 476.9 and − 200.8 cal/mole, respectively.

(b) The absorbance of the complex calculated from the Benesi − Hildebrand equation is:

$$\frac{0.02}{A} = \frac{1}{66} + \frac{1}{(66)(3.5)(0.5)} = 0.024; \quad A = 0.833 \text{ at } 5°C.$$

PROBLEM 11.13. A plot of $\frac{1}{\Delta^A_{obs}}$

versus $\frac{1}{C_D}$ (Figure P11-3) gives the apparent

stability constant from the slope. The complexation shift is given from the intercept. Or, more accurately, these constants can be

obtained from a regression of $\frac{1}{\Delta^A_{obs}}$ against $\frac{1}{C_D}$.

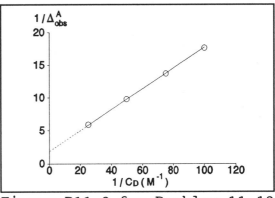

Figure P11-3 for Problem 11.13

By least squares, the equation is found to be:

$$\frac{1}{\Delta^A_{obs}} = 0.156 \frac{1}{C_D} + 2.00 ; \quad \text{Intercept} = 2.00 = \frac{1}{(\delta^A_c - \delta^A_m)}; \quad (\delta^A_c - \delta^A_m) = 0.50$$

Slope, $0.156 = \frac{1}{K(\delta^A_c - \delta^A_m)}$; $K = 1/(0.156)(0.50) = 12.8$

Table P11−5 for Problem 11.14.

% EtOH	ΔG°		ΔH°	ΔS°
	25°C	35°C		
2.5	−5.88	−6.00	−2.38	+11.8
5.0	−5.85	−5.97	−2.30	+11.9
10.0	−5.81	−5.93	−2.15	+12.3
20.0	−5.73	−5.85	−2.19	+11.9

PROBLEM 11.14. (a) For 2.5% ethanol at 25°C, $\Delta G^\circ = -RT \ln K$
$= -(1.9872)(298.15)\ln(20.5 \times 10^3) = -5882$ cal/mole $= -5.9$ kcal/mole

ΔH° is computed from $\ln \dfrac{K_2}{K_1} = \dfrac{\Delta H^\circ}{R}\left(\dfrac{T_2 - T_1}{T_2 T_1}\right)$

At the two temperatures of 25°C ($T_1 = 298.15$°K) and 35°C ($T_2 = 303.15$°K), $K_1 = 20.5 \times 10^3$ and $K_2 = 18.0 \times 10^3$:

$\ln(18 \times 10^3) - \ln(20.5 \times 10^3) = \dfrac{\Delta H^\circ}{1.9872}\left(\dfrac{308.15 - 298.15}{308.15 \times 298.15}\right)$; solving for ΔH°,

$\Delta H^\circ = -2375.9$ cal/mole or -2.4 kcal/mole. ΔS° at 25°C is calculated from

$\Delta S^\circ = \dfrac{\Delta H^\circ - \Delta G^\circ}{T} = \dfrac{-2375.9 + 5882}{298.15} = +11.8$ cal/(mole deg). Similarly, the

results for each mixture are found in Table P11−5. The values of ΔG° and ΔH° are given in kcal/mole, and the values of ΔS° are in cal/(mole deg).

(b) A plot of the thermodynamics values obtained is shown in Figure P11−4.

(c) The positive entropy may be the result of <u>hydrophobic</u> <u>interaction</u> that squeezes out the water molecules surrounding the polymer and the drug. The complex formed may be

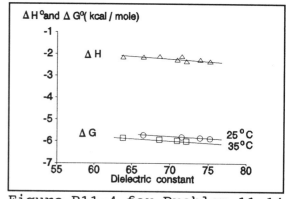

Figure P11-4 for Problem 11.14

acompanied by an iceberg which is less ordered than the icebergs of the two separate entities, resulting in an increase of entropy. The associaton constants, K, decrease and ΔG° becomes less negative as the dielectric constant decreases. The reaction is exothermic for all mixtures (negative ΔH°). This could indicate hydrogen bonding or van der Waals interaction forces. If one assumes that ΔH° for hydrogen bonding is about -5 kcal/mole, substracting this value from the calculated ΔH° for any of the mixtures, results in a positive enthalpy value. For example, for the 2.5% ethanol mixture, one obtains -2.4 kcal/mole $- (-5$ kcal/mole) $= +2.6$ kcal/mole. This positive enthalpy value , together with the positive entropies obtained, correspond to hydrophobic interaction. (See the paper by J. A. Plaizier – Vercammen and R. E. De Neve, J. Pharm. Sci., $\underline{71}$, 552, 1982, for a detailed discussion on the thermodynamics of the process).

PROBLEM 11.15. (a) The Scatchard plot is shown in Figure P11 – 5. Using linear regression, one obtains

$$\frac{r}{[D]} = 0.15168 - 0.05519 \ r.$$

The association constant K is obtained from the slope:

$(-\text{slope}) = K = 0.05519 \ \text{L}/\mu\text{mole}$

$= 55,190$ L/mole.

The number of binding ν sites is computed from the intercept:

Figure P11-5 for Problem 11.15

Intercept $= K \ \nu$, and $\nu = \dfrac{intercept}{K} = \dfrac{0.15168}{0.05519} = 2.75.$

(b) When the concentration of protein is unknown, we use equation (11 – 41). The data needed are shown in Table P11 – 6, where [PD] is the concentration of bound drug and $[D_f]$ is the concentration of free drug.

Table P11 – 6 for Problem 1.15.

$[PD]/[D_f]$	3.03	2.78	1.76	0.91
[PD]	9.1	17.8	30.2	46.1

A regression of [PD]/[D$_f$] against [PD], equation (11-32) gives the results:

$$\frac{[PD]}{[D_f]} = -0.0602 \,[PD] + 3.6735$$

$-$(Slope) $= K = 0.0602$ L/μmole $= 60,200$ L/mole; this value is close enough to that obtained in part (a), 55,190 L/mole.

The amount of protein can be computed from the intercept.

Intercept $= 3.6735 = \nu K(P_t)$; using the value $\nu = 2.75$ from part (a),

$$P_t = \frac{3.6735}{(0.0602)(2.75)} = 22.2 \,\mu mole/L.$$

The author obtained a concentration of protein of 23.2 μmole/liter.

PROBLEM 11.16. Inside the sac, there is 0.7×10^{-4} M of caffeine free + caffeine bound; outside, 3×10^{-4} M of free caffeine are in equilibrium with 3×10^{-4} M of caffeine free inside the sac.

Therefore, the amount of caffeine bound inside the sac is (0.7×10^{-4}) M $-$ (0.3×10^{-4}) M $= 0.4 \times 10^{-4}$ M

$$ß = \frac{[Bound\ drug]}{[Total\ drug]} = \frac{0.4 \times 10^{-4}}{0.7 \times 10^{-4}} = 0.571;$$

$$r = \frac{[Bound\ drug]}{[Total\ protein]} = \frac{0.4 \times 10^{-4}}{2.8 \times 10^{-4}} = 0.14$$

PROBLEM 11.17. We express [D$_f$] in mole/liter because the constants K_1 and K_2 are given in these units. For example, for [D$_f$] $= 1.43 \times 10^{-3}$ mM/liter, we use 1.43×10^{-6} mole/liter (M). Using this value and ν_1, ν_2, K_1 and K_2 given in this problem, we compute the value of r:

$$r = \frac{(2.26)\,(1.32 \times 10^5\ M^{-1})\,(1.43 \times 10^{-6}\ M)}{1 + (1.32 \times 10^5\ M^{-1})\,(1.43 \times 10^{-6}\ M)} +$$

$$\frac{(10.20)\,(3.71 \times 10^3\ M^{-1})\,(1.43 \times 10^{-6}\ M)}{1 + (3.71 \times 10^3\ M^{-1})\,(1.43 \times 10^{-6}\ M)} = 0.41,\ and$$

$$\frac{r}{[D_f]} = \frac{0.41}{1.43 \times 10^{-3}\ mmole/\ell} = 288.6\ liter/mmole.$$

By such calculations, we obtain the results shown in Table P11$-$7.

The Scatchard plot (Figure P11$-$6) is not a straight line because there is more than one kind of binding sites in the protein for the drug, in this case 2 sites.

Table P11 − 7 for Problem 11.17.

$[D_f](mM)$ $\times 10^3$	1.43	4.7	16	63	132.4	303.4	533.2
r	0.41	1.04	2.11	3.95	5.50	7.61	9.00
$r/[D_f]$ mM^{-1}	289	221	131.9	62.7	41.5	25.1	16.9

Table P11 − 8 for Problem 11.18.

$r/[D_f]$ liter/mole	23000	15862	11786	7800
r	0.23	0.46	0.66	0.78

PROBLEM 11.18. A linear regression of $r/[D_f]$ against r (equation 11-40) gives K from the slope and ν from the intercept. The values needed for these calculations are presented in Table P11 − 8.

The equation is

$r/[D_f] = -26821\ r + 28894$;

slope = K = 26,821 liter/mole;

intercept = νK

$\nu = \dfrac{28894}{26821} = 1.08$. Therefore there is one binding site, and a Scatchard plot would show a straight line.

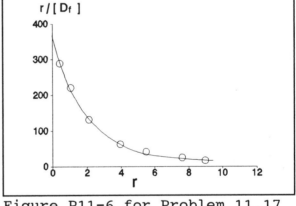

Figure P11-6 for Problem 11.17

PROBLEM 11.19. In case I the concentration, $[D_f] = A/\epsilon b$, of unbound acetaminophen in the absence of phenylbutazone, $[D_f'] = 0$, is

$[D_f] = \dfrac{0.683}{(2.3 \times 10^3)\ (1)} = 2.97 \times 10^{-4}$ mole/liter.

The concentration of bound acetaminophen is $[D_b] = [D_t] - [D_f]$

$= (3.97 \times 10^{-4}) - (2.97 \times 10^{-4}) = 1 \times 10^{-4}$ mole/liter.

Table P11 – 9 for Problem 11.19.

	I	II	III	IV
r	0.17	0.10	0.08	0.07
% bound	25%	14%	12%	10.8%
r (% decrease)	–	41%	53%	59%

$$r = \frac{[D_b]}{[P_t]} = \frac{1 \times 10^{-4}}{5.8 \times 10^{-4}} = 0.17.$$

The percent bound is $\left(\frac{D_b}{D_t}\right) \times 100 = \frac{1 \times 10^{-4}}{3.97 \times 10^{-4}} \times 100 = 25\%.$

For case *II*, the concentration, $[D_f] = A/\epsilon b$, of unbound acetaminophen in the presence of phenylbutazone, $[D_f'] = 0.65 \times 10^{-4}$, is

$$[D_f] = \frac{0.782}{(2.3 \times 10^3)(1)} = 3.4 \times 10^{-4} \text{ mole/liter.}$$

The concentration of bound acetaminophen is

$[D_b] = (D_t) - [D_f] = (3.97 \times 10^{-4}) - (3.4 \times 10^{-4}) = 0.57 \times 10^{-4}$ mole/liter.

$$r = \frac{[D_b]}{[P_t]} = \frac{0.57 \times 10^{-5}}{5.8 \times 10^{-4}} = 0.10.$$

The percent bound is $\left(\frac{D_b}{D_t}\right) \times 100 = \frac{0.57 \times 10^{-4}}{3.97 \times 10^{-4}} \times 100 = 14\ \%.$

The values of r and percent of acetaminophen bound for cases *III* and *IV* are calculated in the same way. Table P11 – 9 shows the results. The entries in the third row show the percent decrease in r *II*, r *III* and r *IV* in reference to the r value of case *I*, i.e. in the absence of phenylbutazone.

For example, % decrease of r *II* $= \frac{0.17 - 0.10}{0.17} \times 100 = 41\%.$ (Table P11 – 9). Thus

we see the competitive effect that phenylbutazone has on the binding of acetaminophen to HSA. See Protein Binding, Chapter 11 of the text, *Physical Pharmacy*, for the competitive effect of one drug on another in their binding to plasma proteins.

PROBLEM 11.20. $k = \frac{\ln(0.27 \times 10^{-3}) - \ln(0.74 \times 10^{-3})}{4 - 2} = 0.500 \text{ hr}^{-1}.$

From equation (11 – 46), at t = 1 hr,

$$\frac{d[D_t]}{dt} = k[D_f] = (1 \times 10^{-3})(0.2)e^{-(0.2)(1)}$$

$$+ (6 \times 10^{-4})(0.1)e^{-(0.1)(1)}$$

$$+ (4 \times 10^{-4})(0.05)e^{-(0.5)(1)} = 0.000237;$$

$$[D_f] = \frac{d[D_t]/dt}{k} = \frac{2.37 \times 10^{-4}}{0.50}$$

$$= 4.74 \times 10^{-4};$$

$$[D_b] = [D_t] - [D_f] = (1.74 \times 10^{-3})$$

$$- (4.74 \times 10^{-4}) = 1.266 \times 10^{-3};$$

$$r = \frac{D_b}{P_t} = \frac{1.266 \times 10^{-3}}{5 \times 10^{-4}} = 2.53;$$

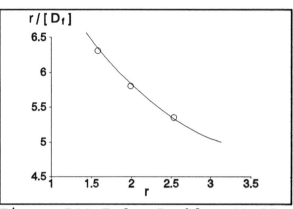

Figure P11-7 for Problem 11.20

$r/D_f = 2.53/(4.74 \times 10^{-4}) = 5.34 \times 10^3$ liter/mole.

Analogous calculations give the results for 3 hr and 5 hr, $r = 1.99$, $r/[D_f] = 5.80 \times 10^3$ (3 hr) and $r = 1.58$, $r/[D_f] = 6.31 \times 10^3$ (5 hr) liter/mole, respectively. The Scatchard plot (Figure P11−7) shows the resulting curve.

PROBLEM 11.21. $\log \dfrac{18}{29} = \dfrac{\Delta H^\circ (303.15 - 273.15)}{(2.303)(1.9872)(303.15)(273.15)}$

$\Delta H^\circ = -2616$ cal/mole

$= -2.6$ kcal/mole; $\Delta G^\circ = -RT(2.303)\log K = -(1.9872)(303.15)(2.303)\log 18$

$= -1741.5$ cal/mole $= -1.74$ kcal/mole.

$\Delta S^\circ = \dfrac{\Delta H^\circ - \Delta G^\circ}{T} = \dfrac{-2616 + 1741.5}{303.15} = -2.88$ cal/mole deg

The negative ΔS° and ΔH° values suggest that hydrogen bonding or donor − acceptor interaction predominates (see Table 11 − 11, Chapter 11). T. Higuchi and D. A. Zuck, J. Am. Pharm. Assoc., <u>42</u>, 132, 1953, also attribute the interaction to a secondary and weaker phenomena involving the nonpolar part of the molecule (hydrophobic interaction).

PROBLEM 11.22. **(a)** and **(b)** Figures P11 − 8 and P11 − 9 show the Scatchard and Langmuir plots, respectively.

(c) Extrapolation to the x − axis of the first linear portion in Figure P11-8 gives ν, the

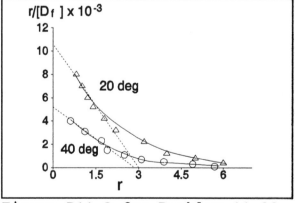

Figure P11-8 for Problem 11.22

first class of binding sites. The values read at 20°C and 40° are about 3, rounded off to obtain an integer.

(d) The slope gives the constant, K, and may be obtained from the two point formula or from regression analysis. Using the five first points and regression analysis:

At 20°C, K = 3.8 x 10^5 liter/mole
At 40°C, K = 1.6 x 10^5 liter/mole.

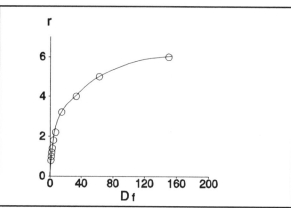

Figure P11-9 for Problem 11.22

These are rough values because the value of the slope obtained either graphically or from regression analysis depends on the number of points chosen. To obtain more accurate values one should use equation (11 – 43), which requires the use of nonlinear regression.

(e) Using the constants obtained by the authors, at 20°C,

$\Delta G° = -(1.9872)(293.15)\ln(3.5 \times 10^5) = -7432$ cal/mole or -7.43 kcal/mole.

The result at 40°C is

$\Delta G° = -(1.9872)(313.15)\ln(1.7 \times 10^5) = -7495$ cal/mole or -7.5 kcal/mole.

(f) $\Delta H°$ is calculated from the data at the two temperatures,

$\ln\dfrac{3.5 \times 10^5}{1.7 \times 10^5} = -\dfrac{\Delta H°}{1.9872}\left(\dfrac{1}{293.15} - \dfrac{1}{313.15}\right)$. Solving for $\Delta H°$ we obtain

$\Delta H° = -6580$ cal/mole or -6.58 kcal/mole.

(g) $\Delta S° = \dfrac{\Delta H° - \Delta G°}{T} = \dfrac{-6580 + 7490}{313.15} = +2.91.$

Analogous calculations give $\Delta S° = +2.91$ e.u. at 40°C.

(h) The binding is a spontaneous process with the compounds in their standard states, because $\Delta G°$ is negative, owing to the negative values of $\Delta H°$ (exothermic reaction) and owing also to the positive $\Delta S°$ values, which represent the change to a less ordered structure. (See the article by M. J. Cho, A. G. Mitchell and M. Pernarowski, J. Pharm. Sci, 60, 196, 1971 for a discussion of the meaning of the thermodynamic functions as related to the binding process).

CHAPTER 12
Kinetics

Table P12 – 1 for Problem 12.1

ln C	− 2.8968	− 2.9356	− 2.9604	− 2.9917	− 3.0407	− 3.0967	− 3.1442	− 3.1917
time, hr	0.5	2	3	4	6	8	10	12

PROBLEM 12.1. If first order, the constant, k, is given by the slope of the plot (Figure P12 – 1). To get an accurate value, we regress ln C against time (Table P12-1). The equation is

ln C $= -0.026\, t - 2.885$; ($r^2 = 0.999$)

$k = 0.026$ hr^{-1}. The half – life, for a first order process is

$$t_{1/2} = \frac{0.693}{k} = 26.8 \text{ hr.}$$ One cannot

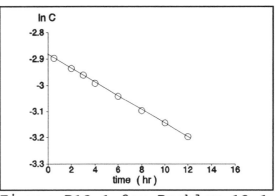

Figure P12-1 for Problem 12.1

determine unquestionably the order from the data, because the times and concentrations given are less than those for 1 half – life. For assurance of the correct order, the data should be recorded for more than 2 or three half – lives (2 or 3 x 26.8 hr).

PROBLEM 12.2. (a) $k_o = k_1[C]$, where [C] is the solubility of ampicillin. Note: 100 ml = 1 deciliter = 1 dl.

$k_o = (2 \times 10^{-7} \text{ sec}^{-1})(1.1 \text{ g/100}) \text{ ml} = 2.2 \times 10^{-7}$ g dl^{-1} sec^{-1}

(b) $t_{90} = \dfrac{(0.10)\,(2.5\ g/dl)}{2.2 \times 10^{-7}\ g\ dl^{-1}\ sec^{-1}} = 1.14 \times 10^6$ sec

1.14×10^6 sec/(86400 sec/day) = 13.2 days.

(c) $t_{90} = \dfrac{2.303}{2 \times 10^{-7}} \log \dfrac{100}{90} = 5.27 \times 10^5$ sec $= 5.27 \times 10^5$sec/(86400 sec/day)

= 6.1 days.

PROBLEM 12.3. (a) The units on the constant, min^{-1} indicate that it is a first order or pseudo first order process. Therefore, the half – life is

$$t_{1/2} = \frac{0.693}{k} = \frac{0.693}{4.863 \times 10^{-3}} = 142.5 \text{ min} = 2 \text{ hr } 22 \text{ min}$$

Table P12 – 2 for Problem 12.3.

t (min)	10	20	30	40
ln C	– 9.8739	– 9.8817	– 9.8896	– 9.8975

(b) Taking ln of C versus time (in the presence of I) we obtain a straight line. The data needed are shown in Table P12 – 2. The constant is obtained from the slope. Using least squares, the equation is

ln C = –9.866 – (7.87 x 10^{-4})t, r^2 = 0.9999.

Slope = k = 7.87 x 10^{-4} min^{-1}; The initial concentration is calculated from the intercept: C_o = exp(–9.866) = 5.19 x 10^{-5}.

The half life is $t_{1/2}$ = $\dfrac{0.693}{k}$ = $\dfrac{0.693}{7.87 \times 10^{-4}}$ = 880.56 min = 14 hr 41 min.

The percent decrease of k is $\dfrac{(4.863 \times 10^{-3}) - (7.87 \times 10^{-4})}{4.863 \times 10^{-3}}$ x 100 = 83.8 %. The

percent increase of $t_{1/2}$ is $\dfrac{142.5 - 880.56}{142.5}$ x 100 = –518 %. (The negative sign means

that $t_{1/2}$ increases in the presence of I).

(c) The concentration after 5 hr (300 min) in the presence of I is

ln C = –9.866 – (7.87 x 10^{-4})(300 min) = –10.102; C = 4.10 x 10^{-5} M, using the equation obtained in part **(a)**.

Without complexing agent, the concentration is

ln C = –9.866 – (0.004863 min^{-1})(300 min) = –11.3249; C = 1.21 x 10^{-5} M. Here, the initial concentration C_o, 5.19 x 10^{-5} M, is that obtained in part **(a)**, and k = 4.863 x 10^{-3} min^{-1} is that given in the narrative of the problem.

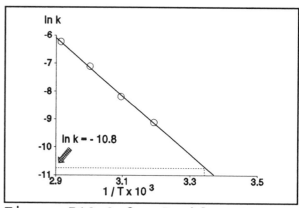

Figure P12-2 for Problem 12.4

PROBLEM 12.4.(a) The data needed for the graph (Figure P12 – 2) are given in Table P12 – 3. From equation (12 – 86), using ln, the slope of the plot obtained graphically, with

equation (1 – 24), slope = $\dfrac{y_2 - y_1}{x_2 - x_1}$, gives $-E_a/R$; this value can also be obtained by

regressing the values in Table P12 – 3. The equation thus obtained is

Table P12−3 for Problem 12.4.

ln k	−9.1150	−8.1807	−7.1062	−6.2348
$1/T$ ($^{\circ}K^{-1}$) x 10^3	3.193	3.095	3.002	2.914

ln k = ln A − $(E_a/R)1/T$; ln k = 24.205 − 10444 $\frac{1}{T}$; r^2 = 0.9987

E_a = −(1.9872)(−10444) = 20754 cal/mole = 20.8 kcal/mole.

(b) Using the equation obtained in part (a), at 25°C (298.15°K), 1/T = 0.003354,

ln k = −(10444)(0.003354) + 24.205 = −10.8242;

k = 1.99 x 10^{-5} absorbance units/hr.

(c) At 25°C, using the constant calculated in part (a), 0.225 = 0.470 − (1.99 x 10^{-5})t; t
= 12311.6 hr ; 12311.6 hr x (1 day/24 hr) = 513 days (1.4 years).

PROBLEM 12.5. Since the initial concentrations are the same, from equation (12 − 23),

$$k = \frac{1}{a\ t}\left(\frac{x}{a - x}\right) = \frac{1}{(0.01)\ (75)}\left(\frac{0.01 - 0.00552}{0.00552}\right) = 1.082 \text{ liter/(mole min)} ;$$

the half−life is

$$t_{1/2} = \frac{1}{a\ k} = \frac{1}{(0.01)\ (1.082)} = 92.4 \text{ min}$$

PROBLEM 12.6. (a) $\quad \frac{d(B)}{dt} = k_3 [AH^+] − k_4 [B]$; if [B] is constant and much less

than [P],

$\frac{d[B]}{dt}$ = 0, and $k_3 [AH^+] = k_4 [B_{ss}]$;

$$B_{ss} = \frac{k_3}{k_4} [AH^+]$$

(b) $\quad \frac{d[AH^+]}{dt} = k_1 [A][H^+] − k_2 [AH^+] − k_3 [AH^+] = k_1 [A][H^+]$

− $(k_2 + k_3)[AH^+]$ = 0 at the steady state; since $[H^+] = [H^+_T] − [AH^+]$,

$k_1 [A]([H^+_T] − [AH^+]) − (k_2 + k_3)[AH^+]$ = 0

Rearranging terms,

$k_1 [A][H^+_T] − [AH^+](k_1 [A] + (k_2 + k_3))$ = 0

therefore, $\quad [AH^+]_{ss} = \dfrac{k_1\ [A]\ [H^+_T]}{k_1\ [A]\ + (k_2\ +\ k_3)}$

(c) Using $[H^+_T] = [H^+] + [AH^+]$ in the final expression obtained in part **(b)**, $[AH^+](k_1[A] + k_2 + k_3) = k_1[A]([H^+] + [AH^+])$; rearranging and canceling terms, we get $[AH^+](k_3 + k_2) = k_1[A][H^+]$;

$$[AH^+] = \frac{k_1 [A] [H^+]}{k_3 + k_2}$$

The rate law is:

$$\frac{dP}{dt} = k_4 B_{ss} = k_4 \frac{k_3}{k_4}[AH^+] \quad \text{(from part (a), } B_{ss} = \frac{k_3}{k_4}[AH^+]\text{)}$$

Using $[AH^+]$ from part **(b)**,

$$\frac{d[P]}{dt} = \frac{k_3 \, k_1 \, [A] \, [H^+]}{k_3 + k_2}$$

PROBLEM 12.7.(a) From equation $(12-53)$, $\ln A = \ln A_o - k_1 t$. The values of k and A_o are obtained from the slope and intercept of a regression of $\ln A$ against t. The data needed are shown in Table P12−4. The equation obtained is
$\ln A = -1.2719 - 0.0383t$ $(r^2 = 0.996)$
$k_1 = $ slope $= 0.0383$ hr^{-1}; $A_o = $ exp(intercept) $= 0.2803$ mM
(b) The calculation of the amount of B appearing as A → B is given by equation $(12-54)$,

$$B = \frac{A_o \, k_1}{k_2 - k_1} \, (e^{-k_1 t} - e^{-k_2 t}) \text{ ; for example, at}$$

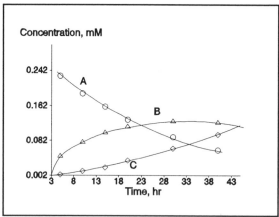

t = 5 hr, A_o is 0.2803 (see part **(a)**)

$$B = \frac{0.2803 \times 0.0383}{0.0243 - 0.0383} (e^{-(0.0383)(5)} -$$

$e^{-(0.0243)(5)}) = 0.046$. The concentration of C is given as $C = A_o - (A + B)$.
A_o was calculated in part **(a)**. Thus, for t = 5 hr,
$C = 0.2803 - (0.23 + 0.046) = 0.004$.
The results for A, B and C are presented in Table P12−5 and are used to construct the plot, Figure P12−3.

Figure P12-3 for Problem 12.7

Table P12−4 for Problem 12.7.

t (hr)	5	10	15	20	30	40
ln A	−1.4697	−1.6607	−1.8326	−2.040	−2.4079	−2.8134

Table P12−5 for Problem 12.7.

t (hr)	5	10	15	20	30	40
A (mM)	0.23	0.19	0.16	0.13	0.09	0.06
B (mM)	0.046	0.079	0.100	0.115	0.127	0.124
C (mM)	0.004	0.011	0.02	0.035	0.063	0.096

(c) For A, $t_{1/2} = \dfrac{0.693}{0.0383} = 18.1$ hr. The concentrations of B and C at this time are

$$B_{(18.1)} = \frac{0.280 \times 0.0383}{0.0243 - 0.0383} \times (e^{-(0.0383)(18.1)} - e^{-(0.0243)(18.1)}) = 0.110 \text{ mM}$$

$$C_{(18.1)} = A_o - \left(\frac{A_o}{2}\right) - B_{(18.1)} = 0.2803 - 0.14 - 0.110 = 0.03 \text{ mM}$$

PROBLEM 12.8. From equation (12−14),

$$k = \frac{1}{10 \ hr} \ \ln \frac{0.05 \ mole/\ell}{0.015 \ mole/\ell} = 0.1204 \text{ hr}^{-1}$$

The concentration after 2 hr, from equation (12−12) is

ln c $= -2.9957 - (0.1204 \text{ hr}^{-1})(2 \text{ hr}) = -3.2365$;   c = 0.039 M

The activation energy is computed from the Arrhenius equation. Using ln,

$$\ln \frac{k_2}{k_1} = \frac{E_a \ (T_2 - T_1)}{R T_2 T_1};$$

solving for E_a,

$$E_a = \left(\ln \frac{0.1204}{0.002}\right)\left(\frac{(1.9872) \ (313.15) \ (293.15)}{313.15 - 293.15}\right)$$

$= 37376$ cal/mole $= 37.4$ kcal/mole.

The Arrhenius factor is calculated from $\ln k = \ln A - \dfrac{E_a}{R \ T}$

ln A $= (\ln 0.0020) + \dfrac{37376}{(1.9872) \ (293.15)} = 57.945$; A $= 1.46 \times 10^{25} \text{ sec}^{-1}$

PROBLEM 12.9. $\ln(1.6 \times 10^{-2}) = \ln A - \dfrac{7700}{(1.9872)(313.15)}$;

$\ln A = -8.2384$, $A = 3.8 \times 10^3 \text{ sec}^{-1}$

The small E_a value suggests that the compound is not highly stable at 40°C.

PROBLEM 12.10.   The data needed for Figure P12−4 are listed in Table P12−6. The E_a value can be mesured graphycally from the slope

of the graph (slope $= \dfrac{y_2 - y_1}{x_2 - x_1}$), or from a

regression of ln k against 1/T. Using the data given in Table P12−6, the equation is

$\ln k = -10217.64 \dfrac{1}{T} + 29.1068$;

$E_a = (-\text{slope})(1.9872) =$
$(10217.64)(1.9872) = 20305 \text{ cal/mole}$
$= 20.3 \text{ kcal/mole.}$
$\ln A = \text{intercept} = 29.1068$; $A = 4.37 \times 10^{12} \text{ hr}^{-1}$
$= 4.37 \times 10^{12} \text{ hr}^{-1}/(3600 \text{ sec/hr}) = 1.2 \times 10^9 \text{ sec}^{-1}$

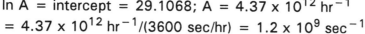

Figure P12-4 for Problem 12.10

PROBLEM 12.11. Using least squares and the data given in Table P12−7:

$\ln k_{OH^-} = 33.4989 - 9071.7 \dfrac{1}{T}$ $(r^2 = 0.9798)$

Intercept $= \ln A = 33.4989$; $A = 3.54 \times 10^{14} \text{ sec}^{-1}$
$E_a = (1.9872)(-\text{slope}) = (1.9872)(9071.7) = 18027 \text{ cal/mole} \approx 18 \text{ kcal/mole}$

Table P12−6 for Problem 12.10.

1/T (°K^{-1} x 10^3)	3.224	3.163	3.057
ln k	−3.835	−3.2114	−2.1286

Table P12−7 for Problem 12.11.

1/T x 10^3	3.354	3.245	3.095	2.832
ln k_{OH^-}	2.7408	4.3567	5.6168	7.6497

PROBLEM 12.12. From regression analysis,

$\ln k = 33.547 - 14974.7 \, \frac{1}{T}; \, r^2 = 0.9998$

$\ln A = 33.547; \, A = 3.71 \times 10^{14} \, hr^{-1}$

$E_a = -(1.9872)(-14974.7) = 29{,}758 \, cal/mole = 29.8 \, kcal/mole$

PROBLEM 12.13.(a) $v = \dfrac{RT}{Nh} = \dfrac{(8.314 \times 10^7)(37.5 + 273.15)}{(6.02 \times 10^{23})(6.63 \times 10^{-27})};$

$v = 6.47 \times 10^{12} \, sec^{-1} = 2.33 \times 10^{16} \, hr^{-1}.$

The gas constant R, is given in erg mole^{-1} deg^{-1}

$\ln A = \ln v + \dfrac{\Delta S^{\ddagger}}{R};$

$\Delta S^{\ddagger} = [\ln(2 \times 10^7 \, hr^{-1}) - \ln(2.33 \times 10^{16} \, hr^{-1})](1.9872) = -41.5 \, cal/mole \, deg$

From equations (12−94) and (12−97) in logarithmic form, $\ln k = \ln A - \dfrac{\Delta E^{\ddagger}}{RT}$,

$\ln k = 16.8112 - \dfrac{12000}{(1.9872)(310.65)} = -2.6275; \quad k = 0.072 \, hr^{-1}$

$\Delta G^{\ddagger} = \Delta H^{\ddagger} - T \Delta S^{\ddagger} = 12000 - (310.65)(-41.5) = 24892 \, cal/mole$

$= 24.9 \, kcal/mole$, where $\Delta E^{\ddagger}$ is approximated by $\Delta H^{\ddagger}$.

(b) $\ln C = \ln C_o - kt = (\ln 0.75) - (0.072)(6) = 0.7197;$

$C = 0.49 \, mg/ml$ of methenamine not hydrolyzed after 6 hours. The concentration of formaldehyde is $C = C_o - 0.49 = 0.75 - 0.49 = 0.26 \, mg/ml$ of formaldehyde formed from methenamine.

(c) The effective concentration of formaldehyde is 20 $\mu g/ml$ or 0.02 mg/ml. Therefore, $C = 0.75 - 0.02 = 0.73 \, mg/ml$ of methenamine remaining.

$\ln (0.73) = \ln (0.75) - 0.072 \, t; \quad t = 0.38 \, hr$ or 22.5 min.

PROBLEM 12.14. The regression analysis of y versus x gives:

$y = 67.968 - 30.993 \, x \quad (r^2 = 0.9875)$

$slope = -\dfrac{E_a}{R}; \quad E_a = (1.9872)(30.993) = 61.6 \, kcal/mole$

PROBLEM 12.15. $\ln k = \ln \dfrac{RT}{Nh} + \dfrac{\Delta S^{\ddagger}}{R} - \dfrac{\Delta H^{\ddagger}}{RT};$

$\ln 0.011 = \ln \dfrac{(8.314 \times 10^7)(313.15)}{(6.023 \times 10^{23})(6.63 \times 10^{-27})} + \dfrac{\Delta S^{\ddagger}}{R} - \dfrac{13800}{(1.9872)(313.15)},$

where R is given as 8.314×10^7 erg/(mole deg) in the <u>first term of the hand side</u> of the equation, whereas R is written as 1.9872 cal/(mole deg) elsewhere in the equation. Solving for $\Delta S^{\ddagger}$ one obtains

$\Delta S^{\ddagger}$ = (1.9872)(22.1776 − 29.0521 − 4.5099) = −23.53 cal/(mole deg).

$\Delta G^{\ddagger}$ = $\Delta H^{\ddagger}$ − T$\Delta S^{\ddagger}$ = 13800 − (313.15)(−23.53) = 21159 cal/mole = 21.2 kcal/mole

PROBLEM 12.16. $\Delta S^{\ddagger}$ is computed from the equation given in problem 12.15.

$$\ln (140 \times 10^{-6}) = \ln \frac{(8.314 \times 10^{7})(370.45)}{(6.023 \times 10^{23})(6.63 \times 10^{-27})} + \Delta S^{\ddagger} \frac{1}{1.9872}$$

$$- \frac{18600}{(1.9872)(370.45)}; \quad \Delta S^{\ddagger} = -26.4 \text{ cal/mole deg}$$

The Arrhenius factor, $A = \frac{RT}{Nh} e^{\Delta S^{\ddagger}/R}$ or $\ln A = \ln \frac{RT}{Nh} + \Delta S^{\ddagger}/R$

$$\ln A = \ln \frac{(8.314 \times 10^{7})(370.45)}{(6.023 \times 10^{23})(6.63 \times 10^{-27})} + \frac{-26.4}{1.9872}$$

$\ln A = 16.3904; A = 1.31 \times 10^{7} \text{ sec}^{-1}$

The probability factor, $\ln P = \frac{\Delta S}{R} = \frac{-26.4}{1.9872} = -13.285; P = 1.7 \times 10^{-6}$

PROBLEM 12.17. The simplest relationship obtained by least squares is:
$\log k_{obs} = 0.111 \delta_1 - 4.504$ ($r^2 = 0.999$)
The logarithm of the hydrolysis rate constant increases linearly with polarity, as shown by the positive relationship. Presumably, the products are more polar than the reactant (maleimide), and the addition of dioxane decreases the polarity of the solvent and protects against hydrolysis. (Figure P12−5).

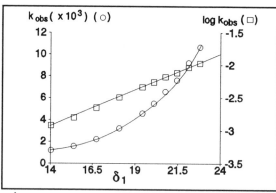

Figure P12−5 for Problem 12.17

However, dioxane is toxic and irritating and cannot be used in nutritive or medicinal products.

PROBLEM 12.18. (a) As shown in Figure P12−6, no kinetics salt effects are observed at pH 2.23 or pH 5.52, indicating that at least one of the reacting molecules, drug or solvent, is uncharged and the slope, $Az_A z_B = 0$ (See Chapter 12, Influence of Ionic Strength). At pH 8.94, the observed k values decrease as $\sqrt{\mu}$ or $\sqrt{\mu}/(1 + \sqrt{\mu})$ become smaller. (Figure P12−6 shows k_{obs} against $\sqrt{\mu}$). Extrapolation of the line graphically gives

Table P12−9 for Problem 12.18.

$\sqrt{\mu}$	0.447	0.632	0.707	0.837	0.940
$\sqrt{\mu}/(1 + \sqrt{\mu})$	0.309	0.387	0.414	0.456	0.487
log k_{obs} (pH 8.94)	−1.6459	−1.5918	−1.5934	−1.5670	−1.5482

$k_o = 0.019$ hr^{-1}.

k_o can also be obtained from the intercept of a regression of log k_{obs} versus $\sqrt{\mu}$ or $\sqrt{\mu}/(1 + \sqrt{\mu})$ (Table P12−9). The equation obtained from regression analysis is

log k_{obs} = −1.7228 + 0.1870 $\sqrt{\mu}$;
$r^2 = 0.9582$
log k_o = intercept = −1.7228;
$k_o = 0.019$ hr^{-1}.

(b) The Debye−Hückel expression for the activity coefficient is

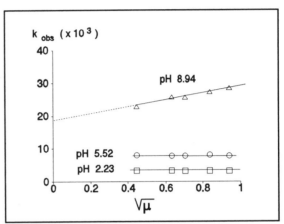

Figure P12-6 for Problem 12.18

$\gamma_\pm = -0.51z^2 \sqrt{\mu}$ in a dilute aqueous solution (< 0.01 M) at 25°C. Solutions here are more concentrated, > 0.2 M, and the corresponding

equation for the activity coefficient is (equation (6−60), Chapter 6) $\log \gamma_\pm = \dfrac{-A z_+ z_- \sqrt{\mu}}{1 + \sqrt{\mu}}$.

The use of this expression should give better results. Thus if we regress log k_{obs} against $\sqrt{\mu}/(1 + \sqrt{\mu})$ at pH 8.94 (data in Table P12−9), we obtain

log k_{obs} = 0.5295[$\sqrt{\mu}/(1 + \sqrt{\mu})$] − 1.8067, $r^2 = 0.9730$
The r^2 value is larger than in part (a), and the slope, 0.5295 is much closer to the theoretical A value, A = 0.51 than the slope obtained in part (a), i.e., 0.187.

PROBLEM 12.19. Plotting k_{obs} versus [H_3O^+], expressed as normality, k_{H^+} is obtained from the slope and k_o from the intercept of Figure P12−7.

Slope = $\dfrac{y_2 - y_1}{x_2 - x_1}$ or $k_{H^+} = \dfrac{0.0115 - 0.0029}{0.0445 - 0.007} = 0.229$

The intercept, read from Figure P12 − 7, is
$k_o = 0.0013$
Using linear regression one obtains
$k_{obs} = 0.001349[H_3O^+] + 0.2276$;
$r^2 = 0.9923$
$k_0 = slope = 0.00135 \ hr^{-1}$

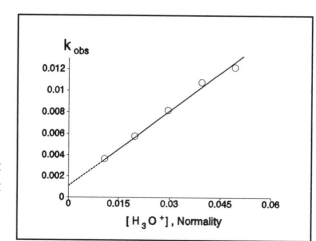

Figure P12-7 for Problem 12.19

PROBLEM 12.20. For compound 7, at pH = 4, $k_1 = 0.024 \ min^{-1}$, $k_2 = 1.8 \times 10^{-4} \ min^{-1}$, $K_a = 6.31 \times 10^{-8}$

$$k = \frac{(0.024)(6.31 \times 10^{-8})}{1 \times 10^{-4} + 6.31 \times 10^{-8}} + \frac{(1.8 \times 10^{-4})(1 \times 10^{-4})}{1 \times 10^{-4} + 6.31 \times 10^{-8}}$$

$= 1.95 \times 10^{-4} \ min^{-1}$.

For compound 8, at pH = 4, $k_1 = 0.42 \ min^{-1}$, $k_2 = 1.7 \times 10^{-3} \ min^{-1}$, $K_a = 6.31 \times 10^{-8}$

$$k = \frac{(0.42)(6.31 \times 10^{-8})}{1 \times 10^{-4} + 6.31 \times 10^{-8}} + \frac{(1.7 \times 10^{-3})(1 \times 10^{-4})}{1 \times 10^{-4} + 6.31 \times 10^{-8}} = 1.96 \times 10^{-3} \ min^{-1}$$

For compound 9, at pH = 4, $k_1 = 2.5 \times 10^{-3} \ min^{-1}$, $k_2 = 0.010 \ min^{-1}$, $K_a = 7.94 \times 10^{-6}$

$$k = \frac{(2.5 \times 10^{-3})(7.94 \times 10^{-6})}{1 \times 10^{-4} + 7.94 \times 10^{-6}} + \frac{(0.010)(1 \times 10^{-4})}{1 \times 10^{-4} + 7.94 \times 10^{-6}} = 9.45 \times 10^{-3} \ min^{-1}$$

Note: The curves for the Mannich bases, no's. 7 and 8 have unintentionally been reversed (Figure 3 in the paper by H. Bungaard and J. Møss, J. Pharm. Sci., *78*, 122, 1989). The open circles are actually the points for compound 8 (not 7), and the triangles are the points for compound 7 (not 8).

PROBLEM 12.21. k_{obs} is obtained from the expression,
$k_{obs} = k_{H^+} [H^+] + k_{OH^-} [OH^-] + k_o$
For example, at pH = 2, $[H^+] = 0.01 \ M$, $[OH^-] = 1 \times 10^{-12}$
$k_{obs} = (2.46 \times 10^{-11})(0.01) + (3.22 \times 10^{-9})(1 \times 10^{-12}) + (7.60 \times 10^{-11})$
$= 7.62 \times 10^{-11} \ sec^{-1}$.
Analogous calculations at the other pH values (4.0, 6.0, 8.0 and 10.0) give the same value, $k_{obs} = 7.60 \times 10^{-11}$ or log $k_{obs} = -10.12$, as shown in Figure P12 − 8, a plot of log k_{obs} against pH. This demonstrates that between pH 2 and pH 10 there is no specific acid − base catalysis. In Fig 1, of the paper by Powell (J. Pharm. Sci., *75*, 9012, 1986), the line is horizontal down to pH = 0, or $[H_3O^+] = 1 \ M$. Below this pH value and above pH 10 the line

begins to curve upward, as shown in Figure P12 – 8. That is, log k_{obs} rises rapidly at strongly acidic medium (pH < 0) and highly basic medium (pH > 10).

PROBLEM 12.22. (a) A plot of log k_{obs} versus pH elucidates whether hydrolysis is due to a specific acid – base catalysis, independent of the nature of buffer and metal added. (Figure P12 – 10).

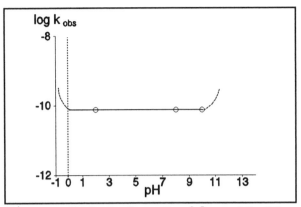

Figure P12-8 for Problem 12.21

The plot shows two slopes one close to – 1.0 and the other nearly + 1.0 as calculated from least squares: (the data needed are found in Table P12 – 11)

Left hand line:

log k_{obs} = – 1.06 pH – 2.25

Right hand line:

log k_{obs} = 0.979 pH – 12.1129

Therefore, neither buffer nature nor metal ions added affects hydrolysis. It is a specific acid – base catalysis.

(b) The constants k_{H^+} and k_{OH^-} are computed from the slopes of the regression equations obtained above as follows. The left hand branch represents acid – catalyzed hydrolysis. According to equation (12 – 123),

log k_{obs} = – pH + log k_{H^+}, where the slope is ≈ – 1, as we found in part **(a)**, i.e.,

slope = – 1.06. The intercept obtained in **(a)** gives

log k_{H^+} = – 2.25, k_{H^+}
= 5.62 x 10^{-3} M^{-1} sec^{-1}

The right hand branch represents the base – catalyzed hydrolysis. According to equation (12 – 130),

log k_{obs} = pH + log k_{OH^-} K_w

where the slope is ≈ + 1, as obtained in part **(a)**, i.e., slope = 0.979.

Intercept = – 12.1129 = log (k_{OH^-} K_w);

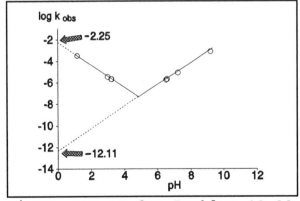

Figure P12-10 for Problem 12.22

Table P12−11 for Problem 12−22.

pH	Data for left−hand branch				Data for right−hand branch			
	1.15	2.99	3.21	3.22	6.51	6.57	7.21	9.22
log k_{obs}	−3.474	−5.456	−5.656	−5.666	−5.730	−5.670	−5.073	−3.078

$k_{OH^-} \cdot K_w$ = antilog(−12.1129) = 7.71 x 10^{-13},

where K_w is 12.63 x 10^{-14} at 80°C.

$$k_{OH^-} = \frac{7.71 \times 10^{-13}}{12.63 \times 10^{-14}} = 6.10 \ M^{-1}sec^{-1}.$$

There is no pH−independent term k_o, representing solvent catalysis in this reaction at the pH range considered. (The points fall on their corresponding straight lines).

PROBLEM 12.23. (a) From the values of the slopes, − 1, 0 and +1, specific acid catalysis occurs between pH 0−4; solvent catalytic effect independent of pH occurs at pH 4−7, and specific basic catalysis at pH 7−10.

(b) pH 6 is within the pH range 4−7 at which catalysis is independent of pH. Therefore, k_{obs} = k_o = 3.064 x $10^{-3} \ M^{-1} \ hr^{-1}$

(c) At pH 8, or [H^+] = 1 x 10^{-8}. Using equation (12−136),
$k_{obs} = k_o + k_{H^+} [H^+] + k_{OH^-} [OH^-]$ = (3.064 x 10^{-3}) + (0.4137 x 1 x 10^{-8}) + (1616.5 x 1.38 x 10^{-6}) = 5.29 x $10^{-3} \ hr^{-1}$

Note: The OH^- concentration is calculated using activities rather than concentrations, see the paper by S. M. Berge, N. L. Henderson and M. J. Frank, J. Pharm. Sci., 72, 59, 1983).

PROBLEM 12.24. First one obtains k_{obs} and plots it against pH (table P12−12 contains the data). Using regression analysis, one obtains

log k_{obs} = 0.8689 pH − 11.150

The slope is nearly +1.0, and the reaction depends mainly on specific base catalysis. (See Figure P12−12).

As shown in problem 12.22 and equation (12−130),

Intercept = log ($k_{OH^-} \cdot K_w$) = −11.15

$k_{OH^-} \cdot K_w$ = antilog(−11.15) = 7.08 x 10^{-12}

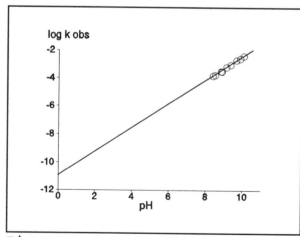

Figure P12-12 for Problem 12.24

Table P12 − 12 for Problem 12 − 24.

pH	8.39	8.51	8.84	8.88	9.13	9.36	9.68	9.89	10.08
log k_{obs}	−3.820	−3.757	−3.481	−3.505	−3.186	−3.031	−2.686	−2.580	−2.392

Table P12 − 13 for Problem 12.25.

1/T (°K⁻¹)	0.00322	0.00312	0.00303	0.00294
ln k	−2.482	−2.198	−1.457	−0.851

$$k_{OH^-} = \frac{7.08 \times 10^{-12}}{10^{-14}} = 7.08 \times 10^2 \text{ sec}^{-1}$$

PROBLEM 12.25. (a) $t_{1/2} = \dfrac{0.693}{k} =$

$\dfrac{0.693}{0.433} = 1.60$ hr at pH = 2. By the same calculations, $t_{1/2}$ for the other pH values are 3.09, 3.73, 8.29, 13.8 hr.

(b) The activation energy can be obtained from the Arrhenius plot (Figure P12 − 13), or

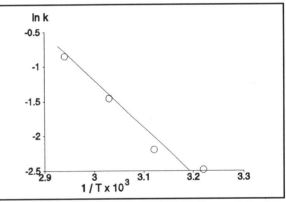

Figure P12-13 for Problem 12.25

can be computed from a regression of ln k against $\dfrac{1}{T}$. The data needed are shown in Table P12 − 13.

The equation thus obtained at pH 5 is

$\ln k = -6004.3 \dfrac{1}{T} + 16.746$

$E_a = -(\text{slope})(1.9872) = (6004.3)(1.9872)$
$= 11.9$ kcal/mole
Intercept = ln A = 16.746;
A = 1.87×10^7 hr^{-1}

PROBLEM 12.26. (a) See Figure P12 − 14.

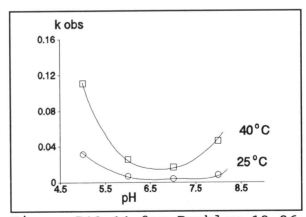

Figure P12-14 for Problem 12.26

Table P12–14 for Problem 12.26.

25°C	pH 5	pH 6	pH 7	pH 8
k	0.0315	0.0069	0.0040	0.0083
$[H^+]$	10^{-5}	10^{-6}	10^{-7}	10^{-8}
$K_w/[H^+]$ $=[OH^-]$	10^{-9}	10^{-8}	10^{-7}	10^{-6}

Table P12–15 for Problem 12.26.

40°C	pH 5	pH 6	pH 7	pH 8
k	0.111	0.0242	0.0169	0.0461
$[H^+]$	10^{-5}	10^{-6}	10^{-7}	10^{-8}
$K_w/[H^+]=[OH^-]$	10^{-9}	10^{-8}	10^{-7}	10^{-6}

(b) The results using multiple linear regression[a] involving 2 independent variables, $[H^+]$ and $[OH^-]$ (see equation 12–150) at 25°C give the coefficients: $k_o = 0.00367$, $k_1 = 2787$ and $k_2 = 4570$ $M^{-1}hr^{-1}$. Thus, the equation is:

$k (25°) = 0.00367 + 2787[H^+] + 4570[OH^-]$.

The k values estimated from this equation are given in Table P12–14.

At 40°C, the coefficients are $k_o = 0.01423$, $k_1 = 9687$ and $k_2 = 11023$ $M^{-1}hr^{-1}$.
The equation is:

$k = 0.01423 + 9687[H^+] + 11023[OH^-]$.

The k values estimated by this equation at 40° C are shown in Table P12–15.

PROBLEM 12.27. The plot of k against $[Na_2HPO_4]$ (Figure P12–15) shows a far steeper slope at pH 6.15 than at pH 6.90

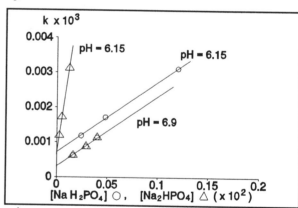

Figure P12–15 for Problem 12.27

[a] Some hand calculators, e.g., Hewlett Packard 41CV, allows one to do multiple linear regression involving two or more independent variables, as needed in this problem.

(although the proportion of [Na_2HPO_4] will be greater at the higher pH). A plot of k versus [NaH_2PO_4] gives almost parallel lines at the two pH's, suggesting catalysis by the same species, $H_2PO_4^-$ at both pH's[a].

PROBLEM 12.28. (a) The expression for the overall reaction is

$k_{obs} = k_{OH^-} [OH^-] + k_1 [H_2PO_4^-] + k_2 [HPO_4^{2-}]$. Since the effect of solvent is negligible, k_o is not included. In order to compute [$H_2PO_4^-$] and [HPO_4^{2-}] at each pH, we use the buffer equation,

$$pH = pK_a + \log \frac{[HPO_4^{2-}]}{[H_2PO_4^-]}$$

where pK_a is the $-\log$ of the second dissociation constant of H_3PO_4. For instance, at pH 6:

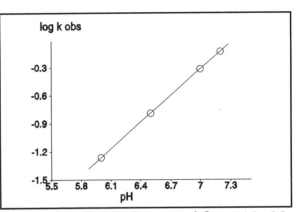

Figure P12-16 for Problem 12.28

$$6 - 7.21 = \log \frac{[HPO_4^{2-}]}{[H_2PO_4^-]} = -1.21; \quad \frac{[HPO_4^{2-}]}{[H_2PO_4^-]} = 0.062$$

Therefore, we have $\dfrac{0.062}{(1 + 0.062)} = 0.058$ moles of HPO_4^{2-} and $(1 - 0.058) = 0.942$ moles of $H_2PO_4^-$ per mole of buffer.

For a total concentration of 0.1 M buffer, we have 0.0058 moles of HPO_4^{2-} and 0.0942 moles of $H_2PO_4^-$ at pH 6. For the other pH values, the results are presented in Table P12-16.

Table P12-16 for Problem 12.28.

pH	6	6.5	7	7.2
$H_2PO_4^-$ (acid)	0.0942	0.0837	0.0619	0.049
HPO_4^{2-} ("salt")	0.0058	0.0163	0.0381	0.051

---

[a] This explanation was provided by Dr. Keith Guillory, University of Iowa.

Table P12−17 for Problem 12.28.

pH	6	6.5	7	7.2
k_{obs}	0.0547	0.162	0.486	0.753
log k_{obs}	−1.262	−0.790	−0.313	−0.123

The total rate constant k_{obs} at pH, say, 6, where $[OH^-] = 10^{-8}$ is:

$k_{obs} = (4.28 \times 10^6 \times 10^{-8}) + (0.036 \times 0.0942) + (1.470 \times 0.0058) = 0.0547 \ hr^{-1}$

Analogously, the other k_{obs} values, as well as log k_{obs} at the several pH are listed in Table P12−17. From these data, a plot of log k_{obs} against pH shows a linear relationship (see Figure P12−16).

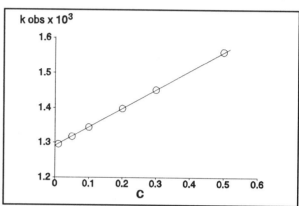

Figure P12-17 for Problem 12.29

PROBLEM 12.29. (a) The plot is shown in Figure P12−17. Since k_o, k_{H^+} and $[H^+]$ are constant, $k_{H_2PO_4^-}$ is calculated from the slope of the graph, and the intercept is equal to ($k_o + k_{H^+}[H^+]$). Using least squares, the equation is

$k_{obs} = (5.40 \times 10^{-4}) [H_2PO_4^-] + (1.29 \times 10^{-3})$.

Slope $= k_{H_2PO_4^-} = 5.40 \times 10^{-4} \ M^{-1} \ sec^{-1}$

(b) From the equation, and using the value,

$[H^+] = 3.16 \times 10^{-4}$ M (pH 3.5).

Intercept $= 1.29 \times 10^{-3} = k_o + k_{H^+}[H^+] = 1 \times 10^{-6} + k_{H^+} (3.16 \times 10^{-4})$;

$k_{H^+} = \dfrac{(1.29 \times 10^{-3}) - (10^{-6})}{3.16 \times 10^{-4}} = 4.08 \ M^{-1} sec^{-1}$

PROBLEM 12.30 (a) Here, the only variable is $[FeCl_3]$. Therefore, the equation is represented only by the first two terms of the general equation given in the formulation of the problem, and the term $k_M'[M][H^+] = 0$. The equation is reduced to

$k_{obs} = k_o + k_M[M]$. (See Figure P12−18). A regression of k_{obs} against [M] gives $k_{obs} = 607.58[M] − 0.027$, $r^2 = 0.994$. From this equation, the slope gives $k_M = 607.58 \ hr^{-1}M^{-1} = 0.169 \ M^{-1} \ sec^{-1}$

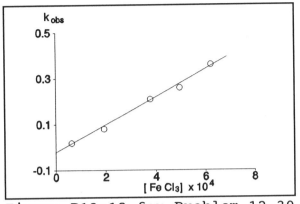

Figure P12-18 for Problem 12.30   Figure P12-19 for Problem 12.30

(b) From the general equation, the term from which we calculate k'_M is the third term. From Figure P12−19, the equation has the form:

k_{obs} = intercept + slope[H^+]

= intercept + k'_MM[H^+]. [M] is incorporated into the slope because it is a constant (6.15 x 10^{-4} M of $FeCl_3$). The intercept is k_o + k_M'[M]. A regression of k_{obs} versus [H^+] gives:

k_{obs} = 0.341 + 1998223[H^+]; r^2 = 0.976

slope = 1998223 = [M]k'_M; k'_M = $\dfrac{1998223}{6.15 \times 10^{-4}}$ = 3.249 x 10^9 M^{-2} hr^{-1} or

9.03 x 10^5 M^{-2} sec^{-1}

PROBLEM 12.31. The first order rate is:

$k = \dfrac{2.303}{20\ months} \log \dfrac{5.0}{4.2}$ = 8.72 x 10^{-3} $months^{-1}$.

For 30% decomposition, i.e., 70 % remaining, the expiration date, $t_{70\%}$, is

$\dfrac{2.303}{8.72 \times 10^{-3}} \log \dfrac{100}{70}$;

$t_{70\%}$ = 41 months. The half life of the product is $t_{1/2} = \dfrac{0.693}{8.72 \times 10^{-3}}$

= 79.5 months.

PROBLEM 12.32. The data needed for the plot are listed in Table P12−18: the inverse of absolute temperature and days to decompose to 80% of the original value. From Figure

Table P12−18 for Problem 12.32.

1/T ($^\circ K^{-1}$) x 10^3	2.75	2.9	3.0	3.1
days	18	43	66	103

P12−20, we read that the drug decompose to 80% of the original value in about 400 days. The method of calculation is explained in Chapter 12, <u>Accelerated Stability Analysis</u>.

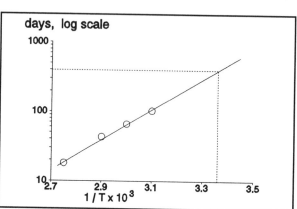

Figure P12−20 for Problem 12.32

PROBLEM 12.33.

$$k_{obs} = \frac{k_f}{k_r} = \frac{0.026\ hr^{-1}}{0.101\ hr^{-1}} = 0.257\ hr^{-1}$$

at 0.04 M concentration of NH_4^+;

$$k_{obs} = \frac{k_f}{k_r} = \frac{0.052\ hr^{-1}}{0.108\ hr^{-1}} = 0.482\ hr^{-1}$$

at 0.08 M concentration of NH_4^+

$k_{obs} = k_o + k_{NH_4^+}[NH_4^+]$; $0.257 = k_o + k_{NH_4^+}[NH_4^+]$ and $0.482 = k_o + k_{NH_4^+}[NH_4^+]$
By solving the two simultaneous equations
$k_{NH_4^+} = 0.225/0.04 = 5.625$ liter/(mole hr); $k_o = 0.032\ hr^{-1}$

PROBLEM 12.34. Since pH has very little effect between $4.3 − 6.2$, the k_{obs} in this range is the k_o which equals 0.056 day^{-1}. Also pH 1.5 converts to $[H^+] = 3.16 \times 10^{-2}$. Substituting these values in the equation, $k_{obs} = k_o + k_{H^+}[H^+] + k_{OH^-}[OH^-]$, and neglecting OH^- at pH 1.5 we get
$0.625 = 0.056 + k_{H^+}(3.16 \times 10^{-2})$; or $k_{H^+} = 18.0\ M^{-1}$ day^{-1}
Now substitute for k_o, k_{H^+} in the above equation and determine k_{OH^-} using the k_{obs} at pH 8.5:
$0.16 = 0.056 + 18(3.16 \times 10^{-9}) + k_{OH^-}(3.16 \times 10^{-6})$;
$k_{OH^-} = 3.3 \times 10^4\ M^{-1}$ day^{-1}

PROBLEM 12.35. First one determines the q values at pH 6.35 and 5.90 using the buffer equation: $pK_a = pH + \log\dfrac{[H_2PO_4^-]}{[HPO_4^{2-}]}$ where pK_a is pK_{a2} of phosphoric acid and

$\dfrac{[H_2PO_4^-]}{[HPO_4^{2-}]}$ is q. At pH 6.35, $7.2 = 6.35 + \log q$, or q = 7.08.

Similarly at pH 5.9, $q = 19.95$.

Since the value of the slope equals $k_2 + k_3/q$ one can set up two simultaneous equations as follows:

$$0.155 = k_2 + \frac{k_3}{7.08} \quad (P12-1)$$

$$0.0556 = k_2 + \frac{k_3}{19.95} \quad (P12-2)$$

Subtracting equation $(P12-2)$ from $(P12-1)$,

$0.0994 = 0.091\, k_3$, or $k_3 = 1.09\ M^{-1}\ day^{-1}$

Substituting this k_3 value in equation $(P12-2)$ yields $k_2 = 0.001\ M^{-1}\ day^{-1}$

The species which catalyzes the reaction is HPO_4^{2-}.

PROBLEM 12.36. $\ln k = \ln A - \dfrac{E_a}{RT}$; at 25°C (298.15°K),

$\ln (0.028) = \ln A - \dfrac{25000}{1.9872} \times \dfrac{1}{298.15}$; $\ln A = 38.61970$

At 70°C (343.15°K),

$\ln k_{70°} = 38.61970 - \dfrac{25000}{1.9872} \times \dfrac{1}{343.15} = 1.95785$; $k_{70°} = 7.08408\ day^{-1}$

$7.08408\ day^{-1} \times (1\ day)/(1440\ min) = 4.9195 \times 10^{-3}\ min^{-1}$

$t_{95\%} = \dfrac{1}{4.9195 \times 10^{-3}\ min^{-1}}\ \ln \dfrac{100}{95} = 10.4\ min$ at 70°C.

Observe the rather large number of significant figures retained in each step of this problem. The calculator or computer is allowed to express each result to the limit of the digits available to the machine. Finally, the answer is rounded off to a reasonable number of digits as ordinarily expressed in problems in kinetics.

CHAPTER 13
Diffusion and Dissolution

PROBLEM 13.1. Using equation (13 − 73), $Q/t = KDC_o/h$

$$Q/t = \frac{6.8\times10^{-3})\,(8.0\times10^{-9}\ cm^2/sec)\,(0.02\ g/cm^3)}{1.40\times10^{-2}\ cm} = 7.77\times10^{-11}\ g\ cm^{-2}$$

sec^{-1}. To obtain the result in micrograms (μg) per day, one must multiply the result by 10^6 $\mu g/g$ and 86,400 sec/24 hour day.

$Q/t = (7.77\times10^{-11}\ g\ cm^{-2}\ sec^{-1})(10^6\ \mu g/g)(86,400\ sec/day) = 6.71\ \mu g\ cm^{-2}\ day^{-1}$

PROBLEM 13.2.

(a) $D = \dfrac{h^2}{6\,t_L} = \dfrac{(0.076)^2}{6\times25} = 3.85\times10^{-5}\ cm^2/hr$

(b) $dQ/dt = DKC_v/h = \dfrac{(3.85\times10^{-5})\,(1.28)\,(0.025)}{(0.076)\,(100)} = 1.621\times10^{-7}\ g/(hr\ cm^2) =$

$1.621\times10^{-7}\ g/hr \times 10^6\ \mu g/g \times 1/cm^2 = 0.162\ \mu g/(hr\ cm^2)$

PROBLEM 13.3. (See Figure P13 − 1)
The regression equations obtained are:
<u>With no binder:</u>
$y = 0.0162 + 0.041\ x$
where $y = \ln(C_s/C_s - C)$ and x is time in minutes.
slope = $k = 0.041\ min^{-1}$
<u>2.5% PVP:</u>
$y = 0.004 + 0.029\ x$
slope = $k = 0.029\ min^{-1}$
<u>5% PVP:</u>
$y = 0 + 0.020\ x$;   slope = $k = 0.020\ min^{-1}$

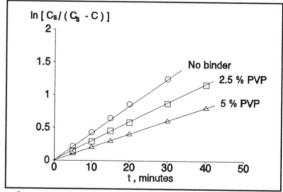

Figure P13-1 for Problem 13.3

Notice that the dissolution rate k decreases as the concentration of binder increases.

PROBLEM 13.4 (a). The data needed for the rectangular and semilog plots, Figures P13 − 2 and P13 − 3, are given in Table P13 − 1. Figure P13 − 4 shows a linear relationship between m and $t^{1/2}$.

Table P13 − 1 for Problem 13.4.

t (min)	2	4	6	8	10	15
$t^{1/2}$	1.414	2.0	2.449	2.828	3.162	3.873
m	14.4	18.8	21.3	25.9	28.2	32.9

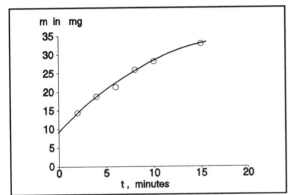

Figure P13-2 for Problem 13.4

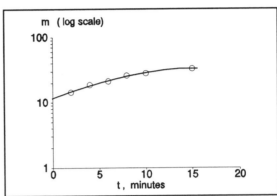

Figure P13-3 for Problem 13.4

(b) The regression equation of the linear relationship (Figure P13 − 4) is:

m = 3.3872 + 7.7055 $t^{1/2}$ (r^2 = 0.9922)

The slope gives the dissolution constant,

k = 7.7055 mg/(min)$^{1/2}$

(c) A possible explanation is that at concentrations smaller than 14.4 mg the curve is not linear.

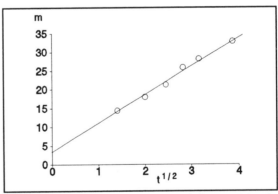

Figure P13-4 for Problem 13.4

PROBLEM 13.5. (a) Using equation (13 − 28) and the value, ($M_o^{1/3} - M^{1/3}$) given in

Table 13 − 6 for t = 2 min, $\kappa = \dfrac{0.080}{2} = 0.04$ g$^{1/3}$/min.

Analogous calculations for the other times give 0.03975, 0.03967, 0.03938, and 0.0396 for t = 4, 6, 8, and 10 min. The average is κ = 0.0397 g$^{1/3}$/min.

(b) A regression of $M_o^{1/3} - M^{1/3}$ against t gives the equation

$M_o^{1/3} - M^{1/3}$ = 0.0394 t + 0.0012,

r^2 = 0.9999. The slope is 0.0394 g$^{1/3}$/min.

This result is very close to that obtained above, κ(av.) = 0.0397 g$^{1/3}$/min. The least squares method is better because it fits the best line to the experimental points. In addition, consideration of the correlation coefficient and regression coefficients allows one to check the agreement of the experimental data with the cube root law. In this case, the agreement is good because r is very close to unity and the intercept, 0.0012 is near zero, as predicted by this law.

PROBLEM 13.6 (a). Equation (13 – 116) is

$$\log R = \log(2.157D^{2/3}C_s a^{1/3}) + \frac{5}{3}\log r$$

According to this equation, the slope should be = $\frac{5}{3}$, and the intercept =

Figure P13-5 for Problem 13.6

$\log(2.157D^{2/3}C_s a^{1/3})$. The data needed are presented in Table P13 – 2. The graph (Figure P13 – 5) shows a linear relationship of log R vs. log r. See Appendix, p. 160.

The equation of the line is (using regression analysis):

log R = – 7.5690 + 1.646 log r

The slope, 1.646, agrees with the theoretical slope, 5/3 = 1.667. The intercept = – 7.5690 compares well with the value $\log(2.157D^{2/3}C_s a^{1/3})$ = log(2.157)[6 x 10^{-6} x 60 cm^2/min]$^{2/3}$(9.4 x 10^{-7} mole/cm^3)(35.066)$^{1/3}$ min^{-1}] = – 7.4739

(b) For r = 1.25, and substituting this value into the regression equation of part **(a)**,

log R = – 7.5690 + (1.646)log(1.25) = – 7.4095; R = 3.90 x 10^{-8} mole/min.

Using the convective diffusion, CD, equation,

R = (2.157)[(6 x 10^{-6})(60)]$^{2/3}$(9.4 x 10^{-7})(3.2731)(1.25)$^{5/3}$ = 4.87 x 10^{-8} mole/min.

The regression equation has an error of about 0.5 % and the CD equation, an error of about 26 % in relation to the experimental value of R = 3.881 x 10^{-8} mole/min.

Table P13 – 2 for Problem 13.6.

log R	– 7.8778	– 7.5667	– 7.4111
log r	– 0.1871	0	0.0969

(c) From equation (13 – 58),

$$h_a = \frac{\pi r^2 D_a C_s}{2R}$$, where πr^2 is the surface area S and R the rate of permeation, dM/dt, and

using the experimental R value of 3.881×10^{-8} mole min^{-1} = 6.47×10^{-10} mole sec^{-1},

$$h_a = \frac{(3.14)(1.25)^2(6 \times 10^{-6})(9.4 \times 10^{-7})}{(2)(6.47 \times 10^{-10})} = 0.0214 \text{ cm.}$$

PROBLEM 13.7. **(a)** $(1.553 \times 10^{-8}) = (2.157)D^{2/3}(9.33 \times 10^{-7}) \times$
$(255)^{1/3}(0.5012)^{5/3}$; solving for D gives us
$D = (0.003848)^{3/2} = 2.39 \times 10^{-4}$ cm^2/min
(b) Figure P13 – 6 shows a plot of log R versus log r. The regression equation is:
log R = $-6.209 + 1.732$ log r. The theoretical slope, 5/3 = 1.667. See Appendix, p. 160.
In a plot of log R versus log C_s (Figure P13 – 7), the slope should be 1.00 since the exponent
of C_s in equation (13 – 116) is unity. The linear least squares equation is:
log R = $-4.556 + 0.991$ log C_s; r^2 = 0.999.

PROBLEM 13.8. $Q/t^{1/2} = [D(2A - C_s)C_s]^{1/2}$

$$Q/t^{1/2} = \left[(3.4 \times 10^{-2}) \left(\frac{2 \times 100 \text{ g}}{10^3 \text{ cm}^3} - \frac{1.50 \text{ g}}{10^3 \text{ cm}^3} \right) \left(\frac{1.50 \text{ g}}{10^3 \text{ cm}^3} \right) \right]^{1/2}$$

= 3.182 g/(10^3 cm^2) per day$^{1/2}$

PROBLEM 13.9.
$Q/t^{1/2} = [(2)(3.4 \times 10^{-2})(100)(1.50)]^{1/2} = 3.194$ g/(10^3 cm^2) per day$^{1/2}$

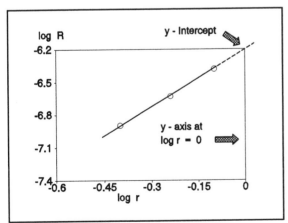

Figure P13-6 for Problem 13.7

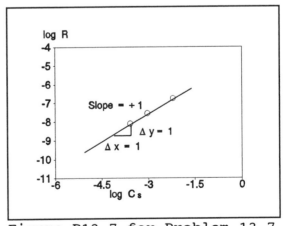

Figure P13-7 for Problem 13.7

PROBLEM 13.10 (a). $2h_a D_m K = (2)(0.003)(2.72 \times 10^{-6})(0.26) = 4.24 \times 10^{-9}$ cm^3/sec; $h_m D_a = (0.0254)(6 \times 10^{-6}) = 1.52 \times 10^{-7}$ cm^3/sec. Therefore, $2h_a D_m K < h_m D_a$ and the process is controlled by the membrane.

(b) When the process is under membrane control:

$$J = \frac{(0.26)(2.72 \times 10^{-6})(60)(1.04 \times 10^{-5})}{0.0254} = 1.74 \times 10^{-8} \text{ mole cm}^{-2} \text{ min}^{-1}$$

Using the entire equation (13 − 59), $J = \left[\dfrac{D_m K D_a}{h_m D_a + 2 h_a K D_m} \right] C_{s'}$

$$J = \left[\frac{(2.72 \times 10^{-6})(0.26)(6 \times 10^{-6})(60)}{(0.0254)(6 \times 10^{-6}) + (2 \times 0.003)(0.26)(2.72 \times 10^{-6})} \right] (1.04 \times 10^{-5})$$
$$= 1.69 \times 10^{-8} \text{ mole/(cm}^2 \text{ min)}$$

PROBLEM 13.11. The flux, is $J = \left[\dfrac{D_m K D_a}{h_m D_a + 2 h_a K D_m} \right] C_{s'}$

$$J = \left[\frac{(0.00972)(10.3)(0.02160)}{(0.006)(0.02160) + 2(0.0188)(10.3)(0.00972)} \right] (1.72 \times 10^{-3})$$
$$J = 9.55 \times 10^{-4} \text{ mmole/(cm}^2 \text{ hr)}$$

PROBLEM 13.12 (a). See Figure P13 − 8.

(b) Using regression analysis of Q against t, the equation is:

$Q = -0.02857 + 0.530t$

The slope is $k_o = 0.530$ mg cm^{-2} hr^{-1}

Intercept $= (D_m C_p/h_m)t_{lag} = -k_o t_{lag}$

$= (\text{slope})t_{lag}$

$t_{lag} = $ Intercept/slope $= 0.02857/0.530$

$= 0.0539$ hr $= 3.23$ min.

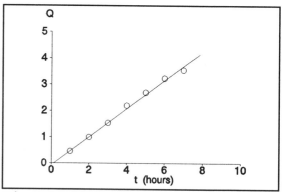

Figure P13-8 for Problem 13.12

(c) Using equation (13 − 14a),

$$D_m = \frac{h_m^2}{6 \, t_{lag}} = \frac{(0.0164 \text{ cm})^2}{(6)(0.0539 \text{ hr})} = 8.317 \times 10^{-4} \text{ cm}^2/\text{hr} = 2.310 \times 10^{-7} \text{ cm}^2 \text{ sec}^{-1}$$

(d) From the slope of the graph and equation (13 − 118),

$$dQ/dt = \frac{D_m C_p}{h_m} = 0.530 \text{ mg/(cm}^2 \text{ hr). Then}$$

$$C_p = \frac{(0.530 \text{ mg/(cm}^2 \text{ hr})(0.0164) \text{ cm}}{8.317 \times 10^{-4} \text{ cm}^2/\text{hr}} = 10.46 \text{ mg/cm}^3,$$

where $D_m = 8.317 \times 10^{-4}$ cm²/hr as obtained in part (c).

PROBLEM 13.13. $\dfrac{1}{P} = \dfrac{h_1}{D_1} + \dfrac{h_m}{\phi \, D_m \, K} + \dfrac{h_2}{D_2 \, K} =$

$$\dfrac{82 \times 10^{-4}}{1.33 \times 10^{-5}} + \dfrac{46.6 \times 10^{-4}}{(0.667)(1.69 \times 10^{-6})(1.16)} + \dfrac{82 \times 10^{-4}}{(1.11 \times 10^{-5})(1.16)}$$

$= 4817.20;\ P = 1/4817.20 = 2.08 \times 10^{-4}$ cm/sec

PROBLEM 13.14 (a). % ionized $=$

$$\dfrac{100}{1 + antilog(pK_a - pH)}$$

At pH say, 4, % ionized $=$

$$\dfrac{100}{1 + antilog(6.5 - 4)} = 0.32\ \%.$$

Percent of undissociated sulfadiazine $=$
100 − 0.3 = 99.7%. Analogous calculations
give the percent of undissociated and
dissociated sulfadiazine at the other pH values
(see Table P13 − 3 and Figure P13 − 9).
(c) In the stomach, pH = 1 − 3, the
nonionized fraction predominates, and the

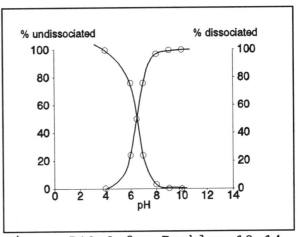

Figure P13-9 for Problem 13.14

drug is easily absorbed. Since the pH in the intestinal tract (pH = 5 − 8) is higher than that
in the stomach, the fraction of nonionized drug is smaller and the absorption is reduced. (see
Table P13 − 3 and Figure P13 − 9).

PROBLEM 13.15. $K_u = 10\ \text{cm}^{-1} \left(\dfrac{2 \times 10^{-4}\ cm/sec}{1 + [(2 \times 10^{-4})/(1 \times 10^{-3})]} \right)$

$= 1.67 \times 10^{-3}\ \text{sec}^{-1}$

Table P13 − 3 for Problem 13.14.

pH	4	6	6.5	7	8	9	10
% dissoc.	0.32	24.02	50	75.97	96.93	99.68	99.96
% undissoc.	99.68	75.98	50	24.03	3.07	0.32	0.040

Table P13-4 for Problem 13.16.

In K (exp.)	0.381	0.026	-0.429	-0.446	-0.574	0.028
In K (cubic)	0.384	0.017	-0.327	-0.561	-0.510	0.017
In K (Davis)	0.579	-0.231	-0.376	-0.362	-0.193	0.187

PROBLEM 13.16 (a). The plot is shown in Figure P13-10.

(b) The squared correlation coefficient r^2 has a value of only 0.784 when carrying out parabolic regression. The cubic equation is better:

$\ln K_p = -0.4541 - 0.3689\,x + 0.2166\,x^2 + 0.0960\,x^3$; $r^2 = 0.957$. The term x in the equation stands for $(\delta_1 - \delta_2)$.

(c) Using the Davis equation (13-120) with the 100% PGE 400 mixture, in which $\delta_1 = 11.8$,

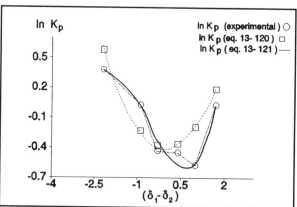

Figure P13-10 for Problem 13.16

$$\ln K_p = \frac{124}{(1.9872)(310)}[(11.8 - 14)^2 - (12.6 - 14)^2] = 0.579.$$

Analogous calculations for the other mixtures give the results shown in Table P13-4 (3rd row), where the calculated $\ln K_p$ values from the cubic regression (2nd row) and the experimental $\ln K_p$ values (1st row) are also recorded.

It is seen from Table P13-4 and Figure P13-10 that the $\ln K_p$ values obtained by cubic regression (2nd row) correspond satisfactory to the experimental $\ln K_p$ values (1st row).

PROBLEM 13.17. (a) See Figure P13-11.

(b) Equation (13-98)(Example 13-14) is:

$P = 4.836 \times 10^{-6} + 4.897 \times 10^{-6} f_B$

where $(P_B - P_{BH^+}) = 4.897 \times 10^{-6} f_b$ and $P_{BH^+} = 4.836 \times 10^{-6}$

At pH 4.67, f_B is 0.01 (see Example 13-14). The permeability calculated from the above

Table P13 – 5 for Problem 13.17.

pH	4.67	5.67	6.24	6.40	6.67	6.91	7.04	7.40
f_B	0.01	0.09	0.27	0.35	0.5	0.64	0.70	0.84
P x 10^6 cm/sec	4.885	5.276	6.158	6.550	7.285	7.970	8.264	8.949

equation is P = (4.836×10^{-6}) + $(4.897 \times 10^{-6})(0.01)$ = 4.885×10^{-6}. The calculated P values at the various pH values, needed for the plot, are given in Table P13 – 5. Figure P13 – 11 shows a plot of P versus pH using the the experimental points from Example 13 – 14 and the calculated line.

PROBLEM 13.18.

(a) Figure P13 – 12 suggests a nonlinear relationship, that can be linearized by taking logarithms on both sides of the equation to give log y = log a + b log x as shown in Figure P13 – 13.

(b) The coefficients a and b of y = ax^b can be computed from the slope and intercept of the relationship written in the form:

log y = log a + b log x

The data needed are recorded in Table P13 – 6.

Using linear regression, the equation is

log y = −0.9554 + 1.005 log x

$(r^2 = 0.919)$

From the equation, slope = b = 1.005; intercept = log a = −0.9554; a = antilog(−0.9554) = 0.111.

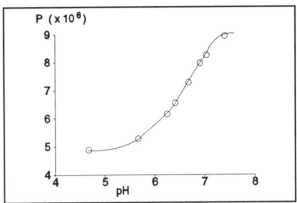

Figure P13–11 for Problem 13.17

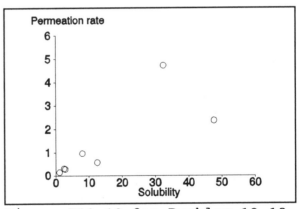

Figure P13–12 for Problem 13.18. See the improvement in this relationship by conversion to a log scale in Figure P13-13.

Table P13 – 6 for Problem 13.18.

log x	0.037	0.391	0.901	0.450	1.097	1.511	1.679
log y	− 0.824	− 0.509	− 0.013	− 0.538	− 0.244	0.675	0.863

The equation is $y = 0.111x^{1.005}$

(c) Assuming a linear relationship between y and x, the equation using least squares is: $y = 0.0724 x + 0.2355$, $r^2 = 0.599$, where slope = $a' = 0.0724$ and intercept = b' = 0.2355. The results of using the power fit are far superior to those of the linear relationship. In the former, 92 % of the variance of log y is explained by log x ($r^2 = 0.911$) whereas in the later only 60 % of the variance of y is explained by x ($r^2 = 0.599$)

(d) From the log – log graph (see Figure P13 – 13), the relationship is log y = log a + b log x, and taking antilogs, $y = ax^b$

(e) Only further experimentation could provide a reasonable answer in response to the hypothesis proposed in (e).

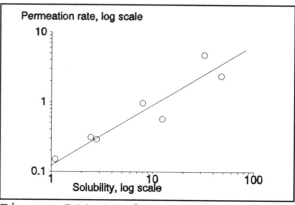

Figure P13-13 for Problem 13.18

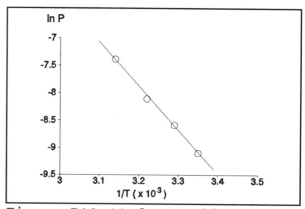

Figure P13-14 for Problem 13.19

PROBLEM 13.19. The data needed for the Arrhenius plot (Figure P13 – 14) are listed in Table P13 – 7. A linear regression of ln P against 1/T using the data from Table P13 – 7, gives the following equation:

ln P = 17.783 − 8023.8 1/T ($r^2 = 0.997$)

Slope = − 8023.8 = − E_a/R.

E_a = (1.9872)(8023.8) = 15945 cal/mole or 16 kcal/mole.

Table P13 – 7 for Problem 13.19.

1/T (°K)	0.00335	0.00329	0.00322	0.00314
ln P	− 9.0970	− 8.5844	− 8.1084	− 7.3858

Table P13−8 for Problem 13.20.

1/T	0.00309	0.00322	0.00330	0.00335	0.00347
ln P	−5.0027	−5.8091	−6.4131	−6.6846	−7.1185

PROBLEM 13.20. (a) The data needed for the Arrhenius plot (Figure P13−15) are presented in Table P13−8. From these data and using regression analysis,

$$\ln P = 12.6150 - 5727.5 \, \frac{1}{T}$$

From the slope, $E_p = (5727.5)(1.9872)$
= 11381.6 cal/mole
From the intercept,
$\ln P_o = 12.6150$, and
$P_o = 3.0 \times 10^5$ cm/min

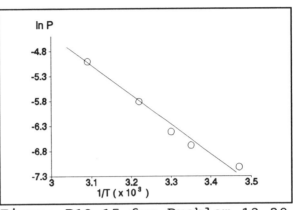

Figure P13-15 for Problem 13.20

PROBLEM 13.21. (a) The values of Q (μmole/cm^2) against t are plotted in Figure P13−16.

(b) From Figure P13−16, J_s (the flux at the steady state) is found, from the slope of the linear segment, to be 15 μmole cm^{-2} hr^{-1}

(c) From equation (13−8), $J_s = (dM/dt)1/S$ so that from equation (13−10b), $J_s = PC_d$; C_d is 1000 μmole/cm^3 or 1 millimole/cm^3.

$$P = \frac{(15 \ \mu mole/cm^2 \ hr) \ (1/60)}{1000 \ \mu mole/cm^3}$$

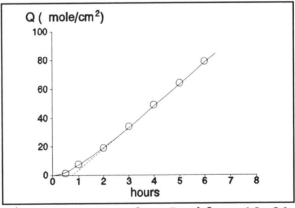

Figure P13-16 for Problem 13.21

= 0.25 x 10^{-3} cm/min.

The term 1/60 in this equation is included to change hours to minutes.

(d) An extrapolation of the linear segment of the penetration curve to zero mass/cm^2 intersects the time axis at $t_L \approx 40$ min (Figure P13−16).

(e) From equation (13−14a), $t_L = h^2/6D$. The barrier thickness h is given as 15 μm = 15 x 10^{-4} cm.

$D = (15 \times 10^{-4})^2/6(40 \times 60) = 1.6 \times 10^{-10}$ cm^2 sec^{-1}

The factor 60 is used to convert t_L in minutes to seconds.

(f) To calculate the partition coefficient K of valeric acid between the skin compartment and the donor vehicle, n−heptane, equation (13−11) is used:

$$K = (P\,h)/D = \frac{(0.25 \times 10^{-3})\,(15 \times 10^{-4})}{(1.6 \times 10^{-10})\,(60)} = 39.1,$$ where the factor, 60 sec/min, converts

seconds to minutes.

(g) Using the equation of Davis, equation (13−125), the ln K is calculated at 37°C. The molar volume of valeric acid is 109.3 cm^3 mole^{-1} and its solubility parameter δ_2 is 9.5. The solubility parameter δ_1 of the solvent, n−heptane is 7.4 and δ_o for the skin barrier, considering it as a hypothetical solvent in which the solute, valeric acid, is dissolved is $\delta_o = 9.7$. V_d, the volume of the applied donor phase, is 300 μL.

$$\ln K = [109.3/(1.9872 \times 310.15)][(7.4 - 9.5)^2 - (9.7 - 9.5)^2] + \ln(300/15) = 3.77;$$
$$K = 43.4$$

PROBLEM 13.22. The constants a, b, and c which are found in the problem, are calculated as follows:

$$a = \frac{1}{2\pi h a_o^2 A} = \frac{1}{(2)\,(3.1416)\,(6)\,(1.1)^2\,(100)} = 2.1922 \times 10^{-4}\ \text{mg}^{-1}$$

$$b = \frac{D_e K_s}{a_o}\left(\frac{1}{P_{aq}} + \frac{1}{P_m}\right) = \frac{(4.5 \times 10^{-7})\,(0.05)}{1.1}\left(\frac{1}{7 \times 10^{-4}} + \frac{1}{5.8 \times 10^{-5}}\right)$$
$$= 3.818 \times 10^{-4};$$

For t = 2.5 days = 216000 sec,

$$c = -2\pi h D_e C_s t = -(2)(3.1416)(6)(4.5 \times 10^{-7})(0.014)(216000) = -0.0513.$$

The amount released at t = 2.5 days is $M = \dfrac{-b + \sqrt{b^2 - 4ac}}{2a}$ mg.

$$M = \frac{-3.818 \times 10^{-4} + \sqrt{(-3.818 \times 10^{-4})^2 + 4\,(2.1922 \times 10^{-4})\,(0.0513)}}{(2)\,(2.1922 \times 10^{-4})} = 14.46\ \text{mg}.$$

Analogous calculations give the values listed in Table P13−9. Figure P13−17 shows a plot of the data.

Table P13−9 for Problem 13.22.

t (days)	2.5	5	10	15	20	25	30	40
m (mg)	14.46	20.80	29.80	36.63	42.44	57.55	52.7	60.37

PROBLEM 13.23.

$$e^{\frac{-\pi^2 Dt}{4H^2}} = e^{\frac{-\pi^2(9.81 \times 10^{-6})(8560)}{(4)(3.92)^2}}$$

$$= 0.986607;$$

$$e^{\frac{-9\pi^2 Dt}{4H^2}} = e^{\frac{-(9)\pi^2(9.81 \times 10^{-6})(8560)}{(4)(3.92)^2}}$$

$$= 0.88572$$

$$R = \frac{(2)(0.0628)}{3.92}(0.986607$$

$$+ 0.88572)[(9.81 \times 10^{-6})(6.780)] = 3.99$$
$$\times 10^{-6} \text{ g/sec} = 2.39 \times 10^{-4} \text{ g/min}.$$

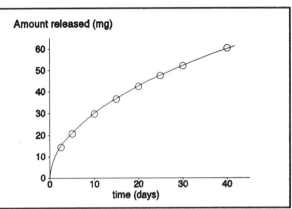

Figure P13-17 for Problem 13.22

PROBLEM 13.24.

$$D = \left[\ln\frac{u - (u_o/2)}{0.5(2u_o/\pi)}\right]\left(\frac{H^2}{\pi^2 t}\right);$$

$$D = \left[\ln\frac{0.0173 - (0.02373/2)}{0.5(2 \times 0.0273/\pi)}\right]\left(\frac{3.86^2}{\pi^2 \times 10523}\right) = 12.4 \times 10^{-5} \text{ cm}^2/\text{sec}$$

where $t = 10523$ sec.

PROBLEM 13.25 (a). From equation (13 – 14b), $P_{dermis} = \dfrac{h}{6 t_L} = \dfrac{0.035}{(6)(152.3)}$

$= 3.8 \times 10^{-5}$ cm/sec

(b) From equation (13 – 51b), the following equations can be written:

$$\frac{1}{P_{whole\ skin}} = \frac{1}{P_{stratum\ corneum}} + \frac{1}{P_{stripped\ skin}} \qquad (P13-1)$$

and $\dfrac{1}{P_{stripped\ skin}} = \dfrac{1}{P_{epidermis}} + \dfrac{1}{P_{dermis}} \qquad (P13-2)$

From equation (P13 – 1), $\dfrac{1}{P_{stratum\ corneum}} = \dfrac{1}{2.98 \times 10^{-8}} - \dfrac{1}{3.74 \times 10^{-6}} = 3.4 \times 10^7;$

P(stratum corneum) $= 3.0 \times 10^{-8}$ cm/sec

From equation (P13 – 2), and the results of part **(a)**,

$$\frac{1}{P_{epidermis}} = \frac{1}{3.74 \times 10^{-6}} - \frac{1}{3.8 \times 10^{-5}} = 2.4 \times 10^5; \text{ P(epidermis)} = 4.15 \times 10^{-6}$$

cm/sec. Note that the main barrier is the stratum corneum, and the most permeable barrier is the dermis.

APPENDIX

In most graphs, the y – axis (vertical axis) is located on the left – hand side of the figure. However, it must be recognized that a graph actually consists of four quadrants, as shown here in Figure P13 – 18. Depending on the sign and magnitude of the independent variable (plotted along the x – axis) and the dependent variable (plotted along the y – axis), the graph of concern may span any one or several of the four quadrants.

Figure P13 – 19 shows the common graph located in the upper right quadrant with its intercept along the upper y – axis of positive values. Figure P13 – 19 also shows the less familiar plot of points occupying the lower left quadrant and having an intercept along the lower or negative extension of the y – axis. The latter is the case found in Figures P13 – 5 and P13 – 6, consisting of the data in Problem 13.6 and 13.7.

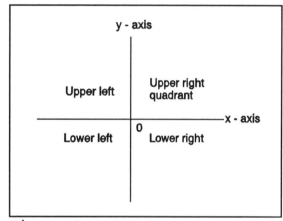

Figure P13–18

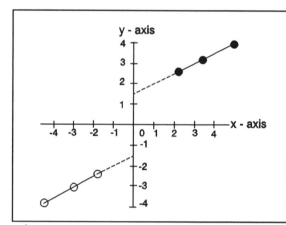

Figure P13–19

Chapter 14
Interfacial Phenomena

PROBLEM 14.1. The hydrogen bonding structure of water is responsible for the high surface tension. When water is heated, the thermal energy partially destroys the hydrogen bonds, and the surface tension decreases. According to Hermann (J. Phys. Chem., 47, 363, 1971), the surface tension of water is due in part to the asymmetric electrical field of the surface layer. Water molecules are randomly oriented in the bulk but at the surface water molecules have their dipoles oriented with respect to the layer below. This results in increased ordering of the molecules at the surface and is the reason for the high surface tension of water. See also M.S. Jhon, E. R. Van Artsdalen, J. Grosh and H. Eyring, J. Phys. Chem., 47, 2231, 1967.

PROBLEM 14.2. (a) $\gamma = \left(\dfrac{1989}{(2)\,(12.47)}\right)(0.920) = 73.37$ dyne/cm; without the

Harkins and Jordan correction, value calculated is $\gamma = \dfrac{1989}{(2)\,(12.47)} = 79.75$ dyne/cm.

The error in the uncorrected value is $= \dfrac{73.38 - 79.75}{73.38}$ x 100 $= -9\%$.

(b) A surfactant will lower the surface tension and improve the spreading of the lotion.

PROBLEM 14.3. γ = force/(unit length) = dyne/cm. If we multiply and divide by cm,

$$\frac{dyne}{cm}\ \frac{cm}{cm} = \frac{dyne\ cm}{cm^2} = \frac{erg}{cm^2} = \text{energy/(surface area), since dyne x cm = erg}$$

and cm x cm = cm^2.

In the SI units, γ = force/(unit length) = newton/m; multiplying and dividing by meter,

$$\frac{newton}{m}\ \frac{m}{m} = \frac{newton\ m}{m^2} = \frac{J}{m^2}$$

PROBLEM 14.4. $\Delta P = \dfrac{2\gamma}{r} = \dfrac{(2)\,(49)}{2.50} = 39.2$ dyne/cm^2

PROBLEM 14.5. $\Delta P = \dfrac{2\gamma}{r} = \dfrac{(2)\,(3.2)}{7.6} = 0.84$ dyne/cm^2;

0.84 dyne cm^{-2} $\dfrac{1}{1.01325 \times 10^6}$ $\dfrac{atm}{dyne\ cm^{-2}} = 8.3$ x 10^{-7} atm

The conversion factor, 1 atm = 1.01325 x 10^6 dyne cm^{-2}, is found in handbooks of chemistry.

PROBLEM 14.6. $\gamma = \frac{1}{2} rh\rho g = \frac{1}{2}(0.02)(6.6)(1.008)(980) = 65.2$ dyne/cm

PROBLEM 14.7. $r = \frac{2\gamma}{h\rho g} = \frac{(2)\,(28.85\ dyne/cm)}{(1.832\ cm)\,(0.8765\ g/cm^3)\,(981\ cm/sec^2)} =$
0.0366 cm radius; 0.0366 x 2 = 0.073 cm diameter.

PROBLEM 14.8 (a). $h = \frac{2\gamma}{r\rho g} = \frac{(2)\,(71.97)}{(0.0023)\,(0.9971)\,(981)} = 64.0$ cm

(b) Capillary action is only a small part of the lifting force of water in trees. The important process appears to be osmosis. As moisture evaporates from the leaves, a concentrated sap remains and water is drawn up through the vascular bundle and across the leaf membranes by osmosis in an attempt to equalize the escaping tendency of water in the tube — like xylem of the vascular tubes and the cells of the leaves. Other processes may also contribute to the rise of sap in trees.

PROBLEM 14.9 (a) $h = \frac{2\gamma}{r\rho g} = \frac{(2)\,(26.99)}{(0.015)\,(1.595)\,(981)} = 2.3$ cm

(b) Knowing γ, r and ρ, it is possible to determine, at least roughly, the value of g. But, see P. Hiemenz, <u>Principles of Colloid and Surface Chemistry</u>, Dekker, New York, pp. 333 – 334.

PROBLEM 14.10. $\gamma = \frac{1}{2} rh\rho g = \frac{1}{2}(0.0230)(2.48)(0.781)(980) = 21.85$ dyne/cm

PROBLEM 14.11. (a) S = 72.0 – 31.2 – 5.7 = 35.10 dyne/cm
(b) The positive sign on S means that the test lotion will spread on a water surface. The instructor might care to have the students survey the literature on the composition of sebum and its possible usefulness as a substrate in such an experiment.

PROBLEM 14.12. Work of cohesion, $W_c = 2\gamma_2 = (2)(25) = 50$ erg/cm^2
Work of adhesion, $W_a = \gamma_1 + \gamma_2 - \gamma_{12}$, where the subscripts 1, 2 and 12 stand for water, organic liquid and water/organic liquid, respectively; $W_a = 72.8 + 25 - 30 = 67.8$ erg/cm^2
Initial spreading coefficient, $S_{initial} = 67.8 - 50 = 17.8$ erg/cm^2

PROBLEM 14.13. $W_c = 2\gamma_2 = (2)(27) = 54$ erg/cm^2
$W_a = \gamma_1 + \gamma_2 - \gamma_{12} = 72.8 + 27 - 8 = 91.8$ erg/cm^2
$S_{initial} = W_a - W_c = 91.8 - 54 = 37.8$ erg/cm^2

PROBLEM 14.14. $W_{SL} = \gamma_L(1 + \cos\Theta) = 63.2[1 + (-0.2250)] = 48.98$ erg/cm^2

In the SI units, 1 erg $= 10^{-7}$ J; $48.98 \frac{erg}{cm^2}(10^{-7}) \frac{J}{erg} \frac{(100)^2 \ cm^2}{m^2} = 0.049$ J/m^2 or,

since 1 J = N m, $W_{SL} = 0.049$ N m^{-1}
$S_{initial} = \gamma_L(\cos\Theta - 1) = 63.2(-0.2250 - 1) = -77.42$ erg/cm$^2 = -0.077$ N m^{-1}

PROBLEM 14.15. (a) The interfacial tension γ_{SL} can be computed from the Young equation, $\gamma_{LV}\cos\Theta = \gamma_{SV} - \gamma_{SL}$; $\gamma_{SL} = \gamma_{SV} - \gamma_{LV}\cos\Theta$
For magnesium stearate, $\gamma_{SL} = 72.3 - (72.8)(-0.515) = 109.8$ dyne/cm; for lactose, $\gamma_{SL} = 71.6 - (72.8)(0.866) = 8.55$ dyne/cm.
(b) $S_{initial} = \gamma_{SL}(\cos\Theta - 1)$; for magnesium stearate, $S_{initial} = 72.8 - [0.515 - 1] = -110.3$; for lactose, $S_{initial} = 72.8[0.866 - 1] = -9.76$
(c) Magnesium stearate has a very high interfacial tension and its spreading coefficient is very negative, so water will not spread over its surface. Lactose has a low interfacial tension versus water, and its $S_{initial}$ value is weakly negative. The contact angle is $< 90°$, and water will wet the surface of lactose more easily than the surface of magnesium stearate.

PROBLEM 14.16. $\Gamma = -\frac{c}{RT}\frac{d\gamma}{dc} = -\frac{5 \times 10^{-3}}{(8.314 \times 10^7)(298.15)}(-32800)$

$= 6.6 \times 10^{-9}$ mole/cm^2. Multiplying the result by the molecular weight, $6.6 \times 10^{-9} \times 107.15 = 7.1 \times 10^{-7}$ g/cm^2

PROBLEM 14.17.(a) See Figure P14 – 1. From a regression of γ against c, the slope is $d\gamma/d(wt\%) = -0.06015$ erg/(cm^2)(wt%)
The intercept is 72.22 dyne/cm.

(b) $\Gamma = -\frac{c}{RT}\frac{d\gamma}{dc}$; for c = 4.96%,

$\Gamma = -\frac{(4.96)(-0.06015)}{(8.314 \times 10^7)(298.15)}$

$= 1.20 \times 10^{-11}$ mole/cm^2
Analogous calculations give $\Gamma = 2.27 \times 10^{-11}$ mole/cm^2 and 3.26×10^{-11} mole/cm^2 for c = 9.34% and c = 13.43%.
(c) For c = 4.96%, $\Gamma = 1.20 \times 10^{-11}$ mole/cm^2, the number of molecules is (1.20 $\times 10^{-11}$ mole/cm^2)(6.023 $\times 10^{23}$ molecules/mole) $= 7.23 \times 10^{12}$ molecules/cm^2; each

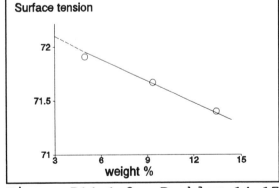

Figure P14-1 for Problem 14.17

molecule occupies $\dfrac{1}{(no.\ molecules/cm^2)} = \dfrac{1}{7.23 \times 10^{12}} = 1.38 \times 10^{-13}$ cm²/molecule = 1383Å². Analogous calculations, using the Γ values obtain in **(b)**, give 730 Å² and 510 Å² for c = 9.34% and c = 13.43%, respectively.

(d) A molecule acting as a surfactant in the surface of water would be vertically oriented and would occupy a space of about 25 to 30 Å². Aminobutyric acid must be lying flat on the surface to take up a space of 500 to 1400 Å² and we conclude that aminobutyric acid is not surface active on water at these concentrations. Of course we could have suspected that aminobutyric acid in these concentrations would not behave as a surfactant in water by an inspection of the table of data. There we observe that the surface tension of pure water is lowered from 71.97 dyne/cm only to 71.40 dyne/cm by the acid in a concentration of 13.43 g/(100 g) of aqueous solution. The molecular weight of aminobutyric acid is 103.12 so the concentration is approximately 1.3 mole/liter of solution. A surface active agent in this concentration would lower the surface tension of water greatly. Both aminobutyric acid, $(CH_3CH_2\ CH\ NH_2)COOH$ and butyric acid, $(CH_3CH_2CH_2\ COOH)$ are completely soluble in water. They do not act as surfactants as do the higher straight chain fatty acids.

PROBLEM 14.18. The limiting slope $d\gamma/d\ln c$ is given by the relationship

$$\Gamma = -\frac{1}{RT}\left(\frac{d\gamma}{d\ln c}\right) \text{ or } -\Gamma(RT) = \left(\frac{d\gamma}{d\ln c}\right)$$

To change Γ in g/m² to mole/m², with the molecular weight of BSA equal to 69,000 g/mole, we write:

At pH 5, $\Gamma = \dfrac{2.54 \times 10^{-3}\ g/m^2}{69000\ g/mole} = 3.68 \times 10^{-8}$ mole/m²

Then with $-\Gamma(RT) = d\gamma/d\ln c$, we obtain at 30° (303.15°K)

$$\left(\frac{d\gamma}{d\ln c}\right) = (3.68 \times 10^{-8}\ \text{mole/m}^2)(8.3143\ J\ ^\circ K^{-1}\ \text{mole}^{-1})(303.15^\circ K) = 9.28 \times 10^{-5}\ \text{N/m}$$

The area per BSA molecule is $A = \dfrac{1}{N\Gamma} = \dfrac{1}{(6.02 \times 10^{23})\,(3.68 \times 10^{-8})}$

= 4.51 x 10⁻¹⁷ m²/molecule = 45 (nm)²/molecule = 4500 Å²/molecule.

At pH 4, $\Gamma = \dfrac{0.70 \times 10^{-3}\ g/m^2}{69000\ g/mole} = 1.01 \times 10^{-8}$ mole/m²

$$\left(\frac{d\gamma}{d\ln c}\right) = (1.01 \times 10^{-8}\ \text{mole/m}^2)(8.3143\ J\ ^\circ K^{-1}\ \text{mole}^{-1})(303.15^\circ K)$$

= 2.55 x 10⁻⁵ N/m

The area per molecule is A $= \dfrac{1}{(6.02 \times 10^{23})\,(1.01 \times 10^{-8})} = 1.64 \times 10^{-16}$ m^2/molecule

$= 164$ (nm)^2/molecule $= 16400$ Å^2.

The conformation of albumin changes with pH so the area also changes. According to Tanford et al. (C. Tanford, S. A. Swanson and W. S. Shore, J. Am. Chem. Soc., 77, 6414, 1955; C. Tanford and J. G. Buzzell, J. Phys. Chem., 60, 225, 1956) there is no configurational change of BSA between pH 4.3 and 10.5. Within this pH range, BSA behaves as a compact, sparingly hydrated sphere. Below pH 4.3, the albumin molecule undergoes reversible transition to a "expanded" form. Tanford et al. (C. Tanford, J. G. Buzzell, D. V. Rands and S. A. Swanson, J. Am. Chem. Soc., 77, 6421, 1955) calculated the radius of BSA at pH 4 from the intrinsic viscosity to give r = 36Å. Accordingly, the area of BSA at this pH value is 4 x 3.1416 x (36)^2 $= 16286$Å^2 or 162.8 nm^2, in good agreement with the calculated value, 164 nm^2/molecule. The maximum radius for BSA found by the authors at more acidic pH values, i.e., between pH 2 to 4, was r = 74 Å, corresponding to an area of 688 nm^2/molecule, or 68,800 Å^2/molecule.

PROBLEM 14.19. $\left(\dfrac{d\gamma}{d\ln c}\right) = -\Gamma RT$

$= -(5.45 \times 10^{-10}$ mole/cm$^2)(8.3143 \times 10^7$ erg/(deg mole))(298.15°K)

$= -13.51$ dyne/cm; area/molecule $= \dfrac{1}{(6.02 \times 10^{23})\,(5.45 \times 10^{-10})}$

$= 3.048 \times 10^{-15}$ cm^2/molecule $= 30.48$ Å^2/molecule

PROBLEM 14.20. From the graph (Figure P14−2), the limiting areas are 0.52 nm^2 (52Å^2) and 0.96 nm^2 (96Å^2) per molecule. The areas are very small, so there is a transition between liquid condensed state and solid state. The gas state or liquid expanded state would show larger areas.

PROBLEM 14.21. Volume = area x length; length $= \dfrac{1 \times 10^{-4}}{400}$ cm

$= 25 \times 10^{-8}$ cm $= 25$ Å

Figure P14-2 for Problem 14.20

PROBLEM 14.22. 1×10^{-4} cm^3 x 0.85 g/cm^3 = 8.5 $\times 10^{-5}$ g;

$$\frac{8.5 \times 10^{-5} \ g}{284.3 \ g/mole} = 2.990 \times 10^{-7} \ mole$$

(6.02 x 10^{23} molecule/mole)(2.990 x 10^{-7} mole) = 1.8 x 10^{17} molecules

$$Area = \frac{400 \ cm^2}{1.8 \times 10^{17} \ molecules} = 2.22 \times 10^{-15} \ cm^2/molecule = 22 \ Å^2/molecule$$

PROBLEM 14.23. Length = $\dfrac{volume}{area} = \dfrac{1 \times 10^{-4}}{250} = 4.0 \times 10^{-7}$ cm = 40 Å

(0.70)(1 x 10^{-4}) = 7 x 10^{-5} g of myricyl alcohol = $\dfrac{7 \times 10^{-5}}{453} = 1.545 \times 10^{-7}$ moles of

myricyl alcohol. The number of molecules is 1.545 x 10^{-7} x 6.02 x 10^{23} = 9.3 x 10^{16}

molecules. The area per molecule is $\dfrac{250}{9.3 \times 10^{16}} = 26.88 \times 10^{-16}$ cm^2 = 27 Å^2

PROBLEM 14.24. M = $\dfrac{RT}{(\pi A/w)} = \dfrac{(8.314 \times 10^7)(292.15)}{2.4 \times 10^6} = 10121$ g/mole

$\approx$ 10,100 g/mole.

PROBLEM 14.25.

M = $\dfrac{(8.314 \times 10^7)(292.15)}{4.02 \times 10^6}$

= 6042 g/mole

PROBLEM 14.26. (a) Figure P14−3 shows the log−log plot. The slope of the line may be obtained from the two point formula. We read from the graph, x/m = 1.259 x 10^{-3} and 1.585 x 10^{-4} at c = 3.162 x 10^{-4} and 3.162 x 10^{-5} respectively, and take the logarithms to get the slope of the line:

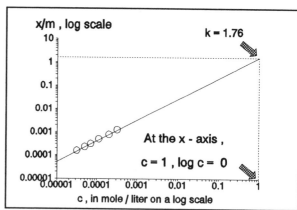

Figure P14−3 for Problem 14.26

1/n = slope = $\dfrac{\log (1.259 \times 10^{-3}) - \log (1.585 \times 10^{-4})}{\log (3.162 \times 10^{-4}) - \log (3.162 \times 10^{-5})}$;

Slope = 0.90 ; n = 1.1

Table P14 – 1 for Problem 14.26.

log c	−4.5000	−4.3000	−4.1500	−3.9500	−3.7000	−3.5000
log (x/m)	−3.8000	−3.6364	−3.5000	−3.3000	−3.1000	−2.9000

The intercept, read at the y−axis at c = 1, i. e., at log c = 0, gives the value of k = 1.76 liter/gram. The units on x/m are mole/gram.

(b) Using regression analysis, n and k are computed from the slope and the intercept, respectively. The data needed are found in Table P14 – 1.

The equation is log(x/m) = 0.9009 log c + 0.2459; slope = 1/n = 0.90; n = 1.1. Intercept = log k = 0.2459; k = antilog(0.2459) = 1.76 liter/gram

PROBLEM 14.27 (a). From the Freundlich isotherm (Figure P14 – 4), using the 2 − point

formula, slope = 1/n = $\dfrac{\log (x/m)_1 - \log (x/m)_2}{\log (c_1) - \log (c_2)}$ = $\dfrac{(0.491) - (0.076)}{1.301 - 0.477}$ = 0.688;

n = 1.45 (dimensionless).

For intercept on the log−log plot (Figure P14 – 4), we read directly k = 0.4 mg/g.

Using regression analysis on the Freundlich log−log equation,

log(x/m) = −0.4048 + 0.6906 log c; r^2 = 0.9999

Slope = 1/n = 0.6906;   n = 1.448 (dimensionless).

Intercept = log k = −0.4048;   k = antilog(−0.4048) = 0.394 mg/g.

The units on k are mg/g because at the intercept, the Freundlich equation requires that c = 1 mg/dl and in logarithmic form, log c = log 1 = 0. Then

log(x/m) = log k + (1/n) log c = log k + 0;   log(x/m) = log k so (x/m) = k and k has the same units, mg/g as has (x/m).

(b) From the Langmuir plot (Figure P14 – 5), using the 2 − point formula,

slope = $\dfrac{1}{y_m}$ = $\dfrac{(c/y)_1 - (c/y)_2}{c_1 - c_2}$ = $\dfrac{6.45 - 3.57}{20 - 3}$ = 0.1694 g/mg;

y_m = 1/0.1694 = 5.903 mg/g.

From the plot (Figure P14 – 5), we read directly the value of the intercept.

Intercept = $\dfrac{1}{b\, y_m}$ = 3.35; $\dfrac{1}{b}$ = 3.35 g/dl × 5.903 mg/g = 19.78 mg/dl;

1/b = 19.78 mg/dl;   b = 0.051 dl/mg

Using regression analysis on the Langmuir equation:

c/y = 1/(b y_m) + (1/y_m)c

c/y = 3.247 + 0.1653 c; r^2 = 0.978

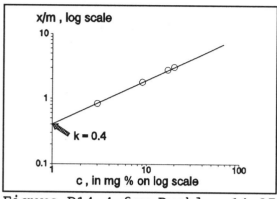

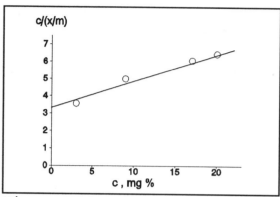

Figure P14-4 for Problem 14.27　Figure P14-5 for Problem 14.27

Slope = 0.1653 (g/mg) = $1/y_m$;　y_m = 6.0496 mg/g

Intercept = $1/(b\, y_m)$ = 3.247 g/dl

$1/b$ = 3.247 × 6.0496 = 19.643 mg/dl;　b = 0.051 dl/mg.

PROBLEM 14.28. Binding capacity = y_m of the Langmuir isotherm = mg of drug adsorbed per gram of activated charcoal or other adsorbent. For a 72 kg patient, 72 g (1 gram for each kg body weight) charcoal is administered.

y_m ×(body weight) = mg of drug adsorbed by the adsorbent, charcoal. For example, for aspirin, 262 × 72 = 18864 mg. The number of tablets is (18864)/(300) = 63. For chlordiazepoxide, 157 × 72 = 11304 mg adsorbed; (113040/25) = 452 tablets. For Diazepam, 136 × 72 = 9792 mg adsorbed; (9792)/5 = 1958 tablets.

PROBLEM 14.29. From the plot (Figure P14 – 6),

slope = $\dfrac{1}{y_m}$ = $\dfrac{(3.4\times10^{-3}) - 0}{(5.3\times10^{-3}) - 0}$ = 0.64;

y_m = 1.56 mg/g;

intercept = $\dfrac{1}{b\, y_m}$ = 0;

b x y_m = ∞; b = ∞

(b) Bone tissues from patients receiving extended doxorubicin therapy were stained. The authors used solid tribasic calcium phosphate as a model to approximate bone tissue samples.

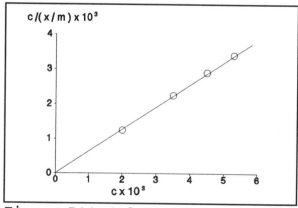

Figure P14-6 for Problem 14.29

Table P14−2 for Problem 14.30.

c	0.5	1	3	5	10	20	50	75	100	110
x/m (37°C)	8.3	14.6	29.0	36.0	47.7	50.6	55	56	56.5	56.7
x/m (50°C)	7.9	13.7	27.2	33.9	41.6	46.9	50.8	51.8	52.3	52.4

PROBLEM 14.30. (a) At 37°C,

$\Delta G° = -RT \ln(102.14)$

$= -(1.9872)(310.15)(4.6263)$

$= -2851.4$ cal/mole $= -2.9$ kcal/mole

At 50°C,

$\Delta G° = -(1.9872)(323.15)\ln(105.457)$

$= -2991.4$ cal/mole $= -3.0$ kcal/mole

(b) $\ln b_2 - \ln b_1 = \dfrac{\Delta H°}{R}\left(\dfrac{T_2 - T_1}{T_2 T_1}\right)$;

$\ln(105.46) - \ln(102.14)$

$= \dfrac{\Delta H°}{1.9872}\left(\dfrac{323.15 - 310.15}{323.15 \times 310.15}\right)$;

$\Delta H° = 490$ cal/mole

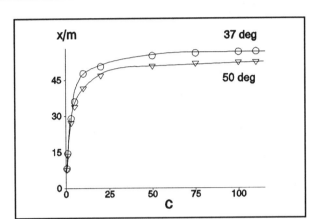

Figure P14-7 for Problem 14.30

(c) At 37°C, $\Delta S° = \dfrac{\Delta H° - \Delta G°}{T} = \dfrac{490 + 2851.4}{310.15} = 10.8$ u.e. By the same kind of

calculations at 50°C, $\Delta S° = 10.8$ u.e.

(d) At 37°C, b = 0.33227 liter/g and y_m = 58.2 mg/g; for c = 0.5,

$x/m = \dfrac{(58.2)(0.33227)(0.5)}{1 + [(0.33227)(0.5)]} = 8.3$ mg/g adsorbent.

At 50°C, $x/m = \dfrac{(53.8)(0.34168)(0.5)}{1 + [(0.3468)(0.5)]} = 7.9$ mg/g adsorbent.

Analogous calculations give the values of x/m at the two temperatures (see Table P14−2). The Langmuir plot for two isotherms is shown in Figure P14−7.

PROBLEM 14.31. (a) The data needed for the plot (Figure P14−8) are listed in Table P14−3. From regression analysis carried out on the equation,

$\gamma = G^s = H^s + \left(\dfrac{\partial \gamma}{\partial T}\right)_P T$ one obtains:

Table P14−3 for Problem 14.31.

T (°K)	293.15	363.15	423.15
γ (erg/cm^2)	63.4	58.6	51.9

$$\text{slope} = \left(\frac{\partial \gamma}{\partial T}\right)_P = -S^s$$

$$= 0.0879 \text{ erg cm}^{-2} \text{ deg}^{-1}.$$

The intercept is 89.60, and $r^2 = 0.981$

(b) H^s is computed at each temperature using

the equation $H^s = \gamma - T\left(\dfrac{\partial \gamma}{\partial T}\right)_P$ with

$$\left(\frac{\partial \gamma}{\partial T}\right)_P = -0.0879 \text{ erg cm}^{-2} \text{ deg}^{-1}$$

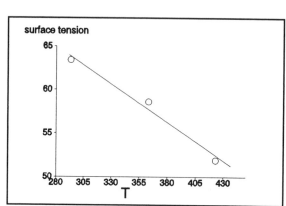

Figure P14-8 for Problem 14.31

At 20°C:

$H^s = 63.4 + (0.0879 \times 293.15)$

$= 89.17 \text{ erg/cm}^2$

Analogous calculations give $H^s = 90.52$ and 89.09 erg/cm^2 for T = 90°C and T = 150°C. H^s is almost constant within this temperature range.

PROBLEM 14.32. The slope, computed from linear regression of γ versus T gives $S^s = 0.113 \text{ erg cm}^{-2} \text{ deg}^{-1}$. H^s is computed using the equation

$$H^s = \gamma - T\left(\frac{\partial \gamma}{\partial T}\right)_P = \gamma + T S^s, \text{ with } S^s = 0.113;$$

At 20°C, $H^s = 26.95 + [293.15 \times 0.113] = 60.08 \text{ erg cm}^{-2}$. At 100°C and 200°C, the H^s values are 59.43 and 60.0 erg cm^{-2}. H^s is almost constant among these temperatures.

PROBLEM 14.33. The data[a] are listed in Table P14−4. Using least squares and the data above between −8°C and 100°C, the equation is:

$\gamma = 120.876 - 0.1647 \text{ T } (r^2 = 0.998)$

slope $= -S^s = 0.1647 \text{ erg/(cm}^2 \text{ deg)}$.

Intercept $= H^s = 120.9 \text{ erg/cm}^2$

---

[a] The instructor may care to assign the calculations at 4 temperatures to each of four groups of students to reduce the labor in this problem. The results of the 4 groups can then be reported and reviewed in class.

Table P14 – 4 for Problem 14.33.

°C	−8	−5	0	5	10	15	18	20
°K	265.15	268.15	273.15	278.15	283.15	288.15	291.15	293.15
γ	77.0	76.4	75.6	74.9	74.22	73.49	73.05	72.75

Table P14 – 4 (Continued)

°C	25	30	40	50	60	70	80	100
°K	298.15	303.15	313.15	323.15	333.15	343.15	353.15	373.15
γ	71.97	71.80	69.56	67.91	66.18	64.4	62.6	58.9

PROBLEM 14.34. (a) $\gamma_L - \gamma_L \cos\Theta = 2\sqrt{\gamma_S^d \gamma_L^d}$; $\cos\Theta = \dfrac{2\sqrt{\gamma_S^d \gamma_L^d} - \gamma_L}{\gamma_L}$

Water – Teflon:

$\cos\Theta = \dfrac{2\sqrt{(19.5)(21.8)} - 72.8}{72.8} = -0.434$; $\Theta = 115.7°$

Analogous calculations for ethylene glycol – teflon and benzene – teflon give contact angles of $\Theta = 92°$ and $50.2°$

(b) From the results, teflon is not hydrophilic and water does not wet it ($\Theta > 90°$). The best wetting agent is benzene ($\Theta < 90°$) followed by ethylene glycol.

PROBLEM 14.35. $\gamma_{o,aq} = 30.8 + 56.9 - 2\sqrt{(30.8)(22)} = 35.6 \text{ mJ/m}^2$

Note that since paraffin oil is a nonpolar substance $\gamma_o^d = \gamma_o$.

CHAPTER 15
Colloids

PROBLEM 15.1. From the graph (Figure P15 – 1), the slope changes when $\sqrt{c} = 0.23$; cmc = $(0.23)^2 = 0.053$ mole/liter.

PROBLEM 15.2. A regression of Hc/τ against τ gives the molecular weight of SDBS from the intercept. See Figure P15-2. The data needed are presented in Table P15 – 1. The equation is

Hc/τ = 0.0147 c + 5.824 x 10^{-5}

Intercept = 1/M = 5.824 x 10^{-5};

$$M = \frac{1}{5.824 \times 10^{-5}} = 17,170 \text{ g/mole.}$$

Slope = 2B = 0.0147;

B = 0.00735 mole cm^3 g^{-2}

Degree of aggregation $= \dfrac{M(aggregate)}{M(monomer)}$

$$= \frac{17,170}{349} = 49$$

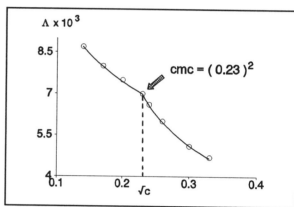

Figure P15-1 for Problem 15.1

PROBLEM 15.3.

$\overline{x} = \sqrt{2Dt}$

$= [2(2.72 \times 10^{-10} \text{ m}^2/\text{sec})(2.30 \text{ sec})]^{1/2}$

$= 3.54 \times 10^{-5}$ meter $= 3.54 \times 10^{-3}$ cm.

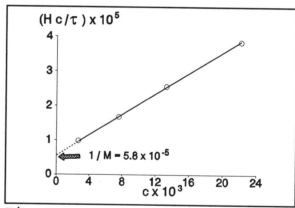

Figure P15-2 for Problem 15.2

Table P15 – 1 for Problem 15.2.

Hc/τ x 10^4	0.983	1.68	2.56	3.84
c x 10^3	2.68	7.58	13.30	22.15

PROBLEM 15.4.

$$\bar{x} = \left[\frac{(8.3143 \times 10^7)(293.15)(3600)}{(3)(3.1416)(0.01)(10^{-4})(6.02 \times 10^{23})} \right]^{1/2} = 3.93 \times 10^{-3} \text{ cm} =$$

39.3 μm or 3.93×10^{-5} meter displacement in 1 hour.

PROBLEM 15.5. The radius may be computed from the relationship $D = \dfrac{k_B T}{6 \pi \eta r}$,

where $k_B = R/N_A$ is the Boltzman constant.

At 20°C, $r = \dfrac{k_B T}{6 \pi \eta D} = \dfrac{(1.38 \times 10^{-16})(293.15)}{(6)(\pi)(0.0097)(7.8 \times 10^{-7})} = 283.7 \times 10^{-9}$ cm

= 28.4 Å. Analogous calculations give r = 54.5 Å, 78.9 Å and 104 Å for T = 25°, 30° and 35°C, respectively.

PROBLEM 15.6. $M = \dfrac{c_g R T}{\pi} = \dfrac{(3.20)(0.0821)(301.15)}{0.00112} = 70{,}641$ g/mole.

(The gas constant R is given as 0.0821 liter atm/(mole deg) and π is the osmotic pressure in atm.

PROBLEM 15.7. The molecular weight of this polystyrene fraction is given from the intercept of a plot of π/c_g against c_g (Figure P15 – 3). To get a more accurate value, a regression of π/c_g against c_g gives:

$\pi/c_g = 6.267 \times 10^{-6} c_g + 8.75 \times 10^{-5}$;

$r^2 = 0.9997$; $M = \dfrac{RT}{intercept}$

$= \dfrac{(0.0821)(298.15)}{8.75 \times 10^{-5}}$

= 279,749 g/mole;

Figure P15-3 for Problem 15.7

$B = \dfrac{slope}{RT} = \dfrac{6.267 \times 10^{-6}}{(0.0821)(298.15)} = 2.56 \times 10^{-7}$ liter mole g^{-2}

Note that the equation is $\pi/c_g = RT(\dfrac{1}{M} + Bc_g + Cc_g + ...)$. We use the Bc_g term, only, in

the expression:

$$\pi/c_g = RT(\frac{1}{M} + Bc_g)$$

UIC company of Joliet, Illinois, makes membrane osmometers for measuring molecular weights in the range of 10,000 to 1,000,000 Dalton. Other methods such as ultracentrifugation and light scattering can also be used.

PROBLEM 15.8. Angular acceleration = $\omega^2 x$ = (6000 rpm x $\frac{2\pi}{60}$)^2(1.2) = 4.737 x

10^5 rad/sec^2; number of "g's" = $\dfrac{4.737 \times 10^5 \ rad/sec^2}{981 \ cm/sec^2}$ = 482.92. That is, the force or

angular acceleration is 483 times that of gravity.

PROBLEM 15.9. From equation (15 – 16), $\omega = \left[\dfrac{\ln(x_2/x_1)}{s(t_2 - t_1)}\right]^{\frac{1}{2}}$ =

$\left[\dfrac{\ln(6.026/5.957)}{(7.756 \times 10^{-13})(15)(60)}\right]^{\frac{1}{2}}$ = 4061.8 rad/sec; $\dfrac{4061.8}{2\pi/60}$ = 38,787 rpm.

PROBLEM 15.10. Angular acceleration = $\omega^2 x$ = (1200 rpm x $\frac{2\pi}{60}$)^2(6.5)

= 102644 rad/sec^2;

number of "g's" = (102644 rad sec^{-2})/(981 cm sec^{-2} = 105 "g"

PROBLEM 15.11. M = $\dfrac{RTs}{D(1 - \bar{v}\rho_o)}$ = $\dfrac{(8.314 \times 10^7)(293.15)(3.6 \times 10^{-13})}{7.8 \times 10^{-7}[1 - (0.75)(0.998)]}$

= 44727 g/mole or 45,000 g/mole.

PROBLEM 15.12.

(a) M = $\dfrac{(8.314 \times 10^7)(293.15)(5.3 \times 10^{-13})}{6 \times 10^{-7}[1 - (0.607)(0.998)]}$ = 54,613 or 54,600 dalton

(b) radius, r = $\dfrac{RT}{6\pi\rho N_A D}$ = $\dfrac{(8.314 \times 10^7)(293.15)}{6\pi(0.998)(6.02 \times 10^{23})(6 \times 10^{-7})}$

= 36 x 10^{-9} cm = 36 Å

PROBLEM 15.13. [η] = KM^a; 2.40 = (4.0 x 10^{-5})M$^{0.990}$, or

log 2.40 = log(4.0 x 10^{-5}) + 0.990 log M;

log M = 4.8264; M = antilog(4.8264) = 67052.5 g/mole

or $[\eta]/K = M^a$; M = $([\eta]/K)^{1/a}$ = $2.4/(4 \times 10^{-5})^{1/0.990}$ = 67052.5 = 67,000 dalton.

PROBLEM 15.14 (a). $[\eta]$ = $(1.1 \times 10^{-3}$ dl/mole$) \times (15200$ mole/g$)^{0.983}$;

$[\eta]$ = 14.2 dl/gram

(b) The units on K in this particular problem are, properly,

$$K = \frac{dl\ g^{-1}}{M^{0.983}(g^{0.983}/mole^{-0.983})} = dl\ mole^{0.983}g^{-1-0.983} = dl\ mole^{0.983}\ g^{-1.983}$$

PROBLEM 15.15.

$[\eta]$ is calculated from the intercept of a plot of η_{sp}/c versus c. The value read at the y−axis is 8.5 (see Figure P15−4).

To obtain a more accurate value, using linear regression, the equation is

η_{sp}/c = 8.526 + 86.4 c (r^2 = 0.9999). The intercept, η_{sp}/c at c = 0 = $[\eta]$

= 8.53 kg mole^{-1}.

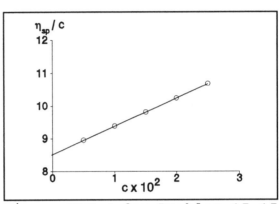

Figure P15−4 for Problem 15.15

PROBLEM 15.16. From equation

$(17-12)$, $\dfrac{\eta_2}{\eta_1} = \dfrac{t_1\rho_1}{t_2\rho_2}$;

$\eta_1 = \dfrac{(614)(1.12)}{(40)(0.997)}(0.01) = 0.172$ poise.

Relative viscosity $\dfrac{\eta_1}{\eta_2} = \dfrac{(614)(1.12)}{(40)(0.997)} = 17.2$

PROBLEM 15.17. $D = \dfrac{RT}{6\pi\eta N}\sqrt[3]{\dfrac{4\pi N}{3M\overline{v}}}$;

$D = \dfrac{(8.314 \times 10^7)(293.15)}{6\pi(0.01)(6.02 \times 10^{23})}\sqrt[3]{\dfrac{4\pi(6.02 \times 10^{23})}{(3)(20,000)(0.9)}} = 11.15 \times 10^{-7}$ cm^2/sec

PROBLEM 15.18. $[\eta]$ = KM^a; taking ln, $\ln[\eta]$ = l K + a ln M

ln M = $\dfrac{\ln[\eta] - \ln K}{a}$. For the experimental intrinsic viscosity η = 0.463,

$$\ln M = \frac{-0.7700 - (-8.21709)}{0.71} = 10.4889, \quad M = 35{,}915 \text{ or } 36{,}000 \text{ dalton. For the}$$

other fractions, the molecular weights are 88,018, 119,940 and 129,342 dalton.

Note: the answers of course will vary somewhat depending on the number of significant figures used in each step. In this problem we retain all significant figures obtained by the hand calculator (10 digits), then round off the answer in the final step. Molecular weights of large molecules are usually given, rounded off to 2 or 3 significant figures.

PROBLEM 15.19.(a) The molecular weight is computed from a regression of $\ln[\eta]$ against $\ln M$ (taking logarithms of the term in the Mark–Houwink equation). The data needed for the regression are given in Table P15–2 and are plotted in Figure P15–5. Note the long extrapolation to obtain the intercept, $\ln K$. The equation thus obtained is

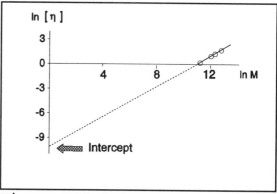

Figure P15-5 for Problem 15.19

$\ln[\eta] = -10.5577 + 0.966(\ln M)$

$(r^2 = 0.9999)$

$\underline{a} = \text{slope} = 0.966;$

$\ln K = \text{intercept} = -10.5577$

$K = \exp(-10.5577) = 2.60 \times 10^{-5}$

(b) For $[\eta] = 7.83$,

$\ln(7.83) = -10.5577 + 0.966(\ln M)$, and $\ln M = 13.0596$;

$M = 469{,}583$ or $470{,}000$ dalton.

PROBLEM 15.20.

$$\zeta = \frac{V}{E} \frac{4\pi\eta}{\varepsilon} = 141\frac{V}{E}; \; \zeta = (141)(25 \times 10^{-5}) = 0.0353 \text{ V} = 35.3 \text{ mV at } 20°C.$$

PROBLEM 15.21.(a) At 25°C, $\eta = 0.008904$ poise

$$\left(\frac{4\pi (0.008904 \; poise)}{78.54}\right)(9 \times 10^4) = 128.2$$

Table P15–2 for Problem 15.19.

$\ln M$	11.125	11.943	12.237	12.704
$\ln \eta$	0.19062	0.97456	1.26413	1.71560

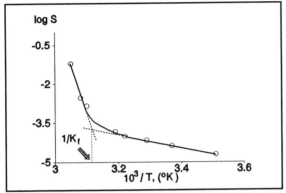

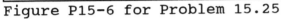

Figure P15-6 for Problem 15.25

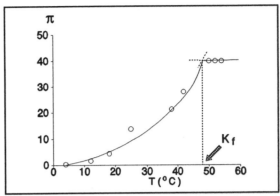

Figure P15-7 for Problem 15.26

At 20°C, η = 0.01002 poise

$$\left(\frac{4\pi\,(0.01002\ poise)}{80.37}\right)(9 \times 10^4) = 141.0$$

(b) ζ for bentonite at 25°C = $(128)(-3.39 \times 10^{-4}) = -0.0434\ V = -43.4\ mV$

and ζ for bismuth subnitrate at 25°C = $(128)(2.20 \times 10^{-4}) = 0.0282\ V = 28.2\ mV$

PROBLEM 15.22.

$$\frac{[D^-]_o}{[D^-]_i} = \sqrt{1 + \frac{[R^-]_i}{[D^-]_i}} = \sqrt{1 + \frac{12.5 \times 10^{-3}}{3.2 \times 10^{-3}}} = 2.215\ \text{to}\ 1$$

PROBLEM 15.23. $\dfrac{[Cl^-]_o}{[Cl^-]_i} = \sqrt{1 + \dfrac{16}{113}} = 1.07$

PROBLEM 15.24. (a) The diffusion coefficient of the micelle in the free solution is calculated from equation (15–3), where the radius is expressed in cm (26 Å = 26 x 10^{-8} cm):

$$D = \frac{RT}{6\pi\eta\, r N_A} = \frac{(8.3143 \times 10^7)\,(298.15)}{6\pi\,(0.089)\,(26 \times 10^{-8})\,(6.02 \times 10^{23})} = 9.4 \times 10^{-8}\ cm^2/sec$$

(b) The intrapore diffusion coefficient, D_p is: $D_p = (9.4 \times 10^{-8})\left(1 - \dfrac{26}{283}\right)^2$

$$\left[1 - 2.1044\left(\frac{26}{283}\right)^2 + 2.089\left(\frac{26}{283}\right)^3 - 0.948\left(\frac{26}{283}\right)^5\right] = 7.63 \times 10^{-8}\ cm^2/sec.$$

Table P15 – 3 for Problem 15.27.

ln n	5.707	5.257	4.956	4.852	4.663	4.357
CP (°C)	42.7	49.7	58.0	64	75.9	107.0

PROBLEM 15.25. From Figure P15 – 6, $1/T = 3.15 \times 10^{-3}$;

Krafft point $= \dfrac{1}{3.15 \times 10^{-3}} = 317.5°K = 43.5°C$

PROBLEM 15.26. From Figure P15 – 7, $K_f = 49°C$

PROBLEM 15.27. One obtains a linear relationship and a positive slope using cmc versus cloud point, CP. With increasing CP the cmc increases. (Figure P15 – 8).

From this relationship one can predict directly cmc from cloud points. The equation of the straight line is cmc $= 9.773 \times 10^{-5}$ (CP) $+ (4.120 \times 10^{-4})$; $r^2 = 0.993$

The aggregation number n is not linearly related to cloud point (Figure P15 – 8). However, trying an exponential relationship like $y = e^x$ or ln y $= x$, leads to a linear relationship. The equation is

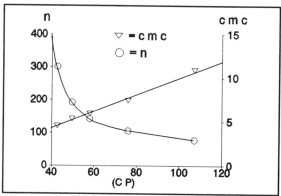

Figure P15-8 for Problem 15.27

ln n $= -0.0187$ (CP) $+ 6.20$; $r^2 = 0.837$. (The data used are collected in Table P15 – 3).The slope of the regression equation is negative: the greater the cloud point, the smaller the aggregation number. Since aggregation number is related to the size of the micelles, the larger micelles will have smaller cloud points; consequently, the solution of the surfactant will separate into two phases at lower temperatures.

PROBLEM 15.28. The maximum value of Γ, the surface excess corresponds to the minimum area per molecule[a],

---

[a] The conversion of units in the equation $\Gamma_{max} = (1/N_A)(1/A_{min})$ may give the student same difficulty. The desired units on Γ_{max} are mole/m^2. We therefore write

$\dfrac{1}{6.02 \times 10^{23} \; molecule/mole} \times \dfrac{1}{49.9 \; Å^2/molecule \times 10^{-20} \; meter^2/1 \; Å^2}$. Cancellation of like quantities yields $\Gamma_{max} = 3.33 \times 10^{-6}$ mole/m^2

$$\Gamma_{max} = \frac{1}{N_A}\frac{1}{A_{min}} = \frac{1}{6.02\times10^{23}}\frac{1}{49.9\times10^{-20}} = 3.33 \times 10^{-6} \text{ mole/m}^2.$$ The surface

pressure π at the cmc is $\pi_{cmc} = \gamma_{water} - \gamma_{cmc} = 71.97 - 36.22 = 35.75$ mN/m.

Finally, $\Delta G°_{ad} = \Delta G°_m - (\pi_{cmc}/\Gamma_m) = -31,800 \text{ J mole}^{-1} - \left(\dfrac{35.75\times10^{-3} \ N/m}{3.33\times10^{-6} \ mole/m^2}\right)$

$= -31,800 - 10,735 = -42,568 \text{ J mole}^{-1} = -42.6 \text{ kJ mole}^{-1} = -4.26 \times 10^{11}$ erg

mole$^{-1} = -10,182$ cal/mole.

PROBLEM 15.29. From equation (15 – A8) of the Appendix, Chap. 15,

$G°_{mic} = (2 - \alpha)$ RT ln (cmc); where $\alpha = Q^-/n$.

$\Delta G°_{mic} = (2 - 0.20)(1.9872)(303)\ln(9.5 \times 10^{-4}) = -7542.35$ cal/mole

$= -7.54$ kcal/mole. Or in SI units, $\Delta G°_{mic} = (2 - 0.20)(8.3143 \text{ J °K}^{-1} \text{ mole}^{-1})(303°K)$

ln $(9.5 \times 10^{-4}) = -3.16 \times 10^4$ J/mole $= -31.6$ kJ/mole.

PROBLEM 15.30.

$$\Delta G° = RT \ln(cmc) = \Delta H° - T\Delta S°; \quad \ln(cmc) = \frac{\Delta H°}{R}\frac{1}{T} - \frac{\Delta S°}{R}$$

According to this equation, $\Delta H°$ can be computed from a regression of ln(cmc) against 1/T. The data needed are found in Table P15 – 4.

The equation thus obtained is ln(cmc) = (469.208) $\dfrac{1}{T}$ – 7.430; r^2 = 0.948

Slope = $\dfrac{\Delta H°}{R}$ = 469.208; $\Delta H°$ = (469.208)(1.9872) = 932 cal/mole

Intercept = $-\dfrac{\Delta S°}{R}$ = −7.430; $\Delta S°$ = (7.430)(1.9872) = 14.76 e u

At 15°C, $\Delta G°$ = RT ln(cmc) = (1.9872)(288.15)ln(0.003) = −3326 cal/mole

The results at the other two temperatures are $\Delta G°$ = −3462 and −3622 cal/mole

Table P15 – 4 for Problem 15.30

ln(cmc)	−5.809	−5.843	−5.915
1/T x 10^3 (°K^{-1})[a]	3.470	3.354	3.245

[a] It is probably less confusing to write the reciprocal temperatures as $(10^3/T)(°K^{-1})$. The first entry in the table is therefore read as 3.470 x 10^{-3} °K^{-1}

Table P15 – 5 for Problem 15.31

ln (cmc) (mole fraction)	− 13.0037	− 13.4253	− 13.5416
1/T x 10³ (°K⁻¹)	3.532	3.354	3.193

PROBLEM 15.31.(a) Using molality units,

$\Delta G°$ (10°) = RT ln (cmc) = (1.9872)(283.15) ln (12.1 x 10⁻⁵) = − 5075.1 cal/mole

= − 5.0 kcal/mole. Analogous calculations give $\Delta G°$ (25°) = − 5.6 kcal/mole and $\Delta G°$ (40°) = − 6 kcal/mole.

(b) The values of cmc are converted into mole fraction:

$$cmc \text{ (mole fraction)} = \frac{m}{\left(m + \dfrac{1000}{M_1}\right)} = \frac{12.1 \times 10^{-5}}{\left(12.1 \times 10^{-5} + \dfrac{1000}{18.015}\right)} = 2.252 \times 10^{-6} \text{ at}$$

10°C. The values of cmc at the other two temperatures are
cmc (25°C) = 1.478 x 10⁻⁶ and cmc (40°C) = 1.315 x 10⁻⁶.

At 10°C, $\Delta G°$ (10°) = RT ln (cmc) = (1.9872)(283.15) ln (2.252 x 10⁻⁶)

= − 7316.9 cal/mole = − 7.3 kcal/mole. Analogous calculations give

$\Delta G°$ (25°) = − 8 kcal/mole and $\Delta G°$ (40°) = − 8.4 kcal/mole.

Table P15 – 5 lists the ln of cmc (mole fraction) needed for the calculation of $\Delta H°$ and $\Delta S°$. $\Delta H°$ and $\Delta S°$ are obtained from a regression of ln (cmc) against 1/T, according to the van't Hoff equation. Using the values given in Table P15 – 5:

ln (cmc) = − 18.700 + 1600.43 $\dfrac{1}{T}$

$\Delta H°$ = slope × R = 1600.43 × 1.9872 = 3180.4 cal/mole = 3.2 kcal/mole

$\Delta S°$ = (−intercept) × R = 18.700 = 37.16 cal/(deg mole).

Micellization is usually controlled by a positive entropy change. The positive sign obtained on $\Delta H°$ and $\Delta S°$ suggests hydrophobic interaction, see Table 11 – 11.

CHAPTER 16
Micromeritics

PROBLEM 16.1. The data needed are listed in Table P16 – 1.

$$d_{ln} = \frac{\sum nd}{\sum n} = \frac{100}{6} = 16.7 \ \mu m;$$

$$d_{vs} = \frac{\sum nd^3}{\sum nd^2} = \frac{46000}{2000} = 23 \ \mu m$$

$$S_w = \frac{6}{\rho \, d_{vs}} = \frac{6}{(1.5)(23 \times 10^{-4})}$$

$$= 1740 \ cm^2/g$$

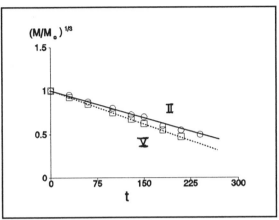

Figure P16-1 for Problem 16.2

PROBLEM 16.2. The data are plotted in Figure P16 – 1. Using linear regression, for sample II,

$$Slope = -2.15 \times 10^{-3} = \frac{(2 \, k C_s / \rho \, f)}{d}; \ intercept = 1.0072$$

$$d = \frac{(2)(0.166)(0.00033)/(1.28)(0.369)}{2.15 \times 10^{-3}} = 0.108 \ cm$$

Sample V: Slope $= -2.5 \times 10^{-3}$; intercept $= 1.000$;

$$d = \frac{(2)(0.166)(0.00033)/(1.28)(0.369)}{2.5 \times 10^{-3}} = 0.093 \ cm.$$

Note in Figure P16 – 1 that in both cases, the intercept = 1. The apparent diameters calculated by the authors correlated well with mean volume diameters and mean weight diameters as determined experimentally.

Table P16 – 1 for Problem 16.1.

nd	nd^2	nd^3
30	300	3000
40	800	16000
30	900	27000
$\Sigma = 100$	$\Sigma = 2000$	$\Sigma = 46000$

Table P16 – 2 for Problem 16.3.

n	d	nd	nd^2	nd^3	nd^4
73	10	730	7300	73000	730000
77	15	1155	17325	259875	3898125
82	20	1640	32800	656000	13120000
37	25	925	23125	578125	14453125
Σ = 269		Σ = 4450	Σ = 80550	Σ = 1567000	Σ = 32201250

PROBLEM 16.3. The data needed are shown in Table P16 – 2.

$$d_{ln} = \frac{\sum nd}{\sum n} = \frac{4450}{269} = 16.54 \; \mu m; \quad d_{vs} = \frac{\sum nd^3}{\sum nd^2} = \frac{1567000}{80550} = 19.45 \; \mu m$$

$$d_{wm} = \frac{\sum nd^4}{\sum nd^3} = \frac{32201250}{1567000} = 20.55 \; \mu m$$

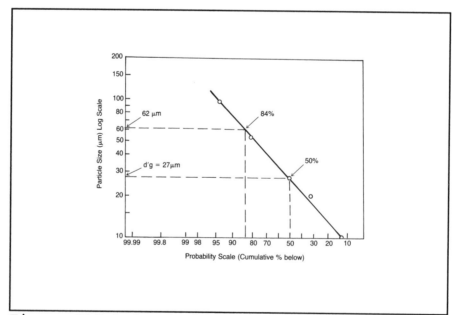

Figure P16-2 for Problem 16.4

PROBLEM 16.4. From Figure P16-2, $d'_g = 27 \ \mu m$.

$\sigma_g = \dfrac{84\%}{50\%};\ \sigma_g = \dfrac{61.9}{27} = 2.3$

$\log d_{ln} = \log d'_g - 5.757 \log^2 \sigma_g = 1.43136 - 5.757(0.36173)^2 = 0.67806;$

$d_{ln} = 4.765 \ \mu m$

$\log d_{sn} = \log d'_g - 4.605 \log^2 \sigma_g;$

$d_{sn} = 6.742 \ \mu m$

$\log d_{vn} = \log d'_g - 3.454 \log^2 \sigma_g;$

$d_{vn} = 9.537 \ \mu m$

PROBLEM 16.5. Using equation (16-6):

$$d_{st} = \sqrt{\dfrac{(18)\ (0.013\ g\ cm^{-1}sec^{-1})\ (6.67 \times 10^{-4}\ cm/sec)}{(3.65 - 1.05)\ g/cm^3\ (980\ g/cm^2)}}$$

$= 2.47 \times 10^{-4} \ cm = 2.47 \ \mu m$

PROBLEM 16.6. $S_w = \dfrac{6}{\rho\,d_{vs}} = \dfrac{6}{(1.5)\ (2 \times 10^{-4})} = 2 \times 10^4 \ cm^2/g$

The conversion factor, $\dfrac{(10^2)^2\ cm^2}{meter^2}$, converts cm^2 to $meter^2$

$S_w = 2.0 \times 10^4 \ cm^2/g \times \dfrac{1\ m^2}{10,000\ cm^2} = 2.0 \ m^2/g$

PROBLEM 16.7. $S_w = \dfrac{6}{(2 \times 10^{-4})\ (2)} = 15000 \ cm^2/g;$

The total surface for 4 g is $= (4\ g)(15000 \ cm^2/g) = 6 \times 10^4 cm^2 = 6 \ m^2$

PROBLEM 16.8. 1 lb = 7000 g; 2000 lb = 1.4×10^7 g

$\dfrac{20\ mg}{1.4 \times 10^7\ g} = \dfrac{x}{40\ g};\ x = 571.4 \times 10^{-7}$ mg antibiotic in 40 grain $= 5.7 \times 10^{-8}$ g in 40

grains of food.
Each 40 grains must contain 1000 particles, so each antibiotic particle weights 5.7 $\times$ $10^{-8}/1000$ or 5.7×10^{-11} g. The volume of each antibiotic particle is

$V = \dfrac{5.7 \times 10^{-11}\ g}{1.2\ g/cm^3} = 4.8 \times 10^{-11} \ cm^3;\ V = \dfrac{4}{3}\pi r^3;$

$$r = \sqrt[3]{\frac{(3)(4.8\times10^{-11})}{(4)(3.1416)}} = 2.25 \times 10^{-4} \text{ cm} = 2.25 \text{ } \mu m. \text{ The diameter is} = 2r = 4.5 \text{ } \mu m$$

PROBLEM 16.9. For the first formulation, $1284 \text{ } \mu m = 1284 \times 10^{-4} \text{ cm}$;

$$SA = \frac{6}{(1.191 \text{ } g/cm^3)(1284\times10^{-4} cm)} = 39.24 \text{ cm}^2/g \text{ or } 39.24 \times 10^{-4} \text{ m}^2/g$$

For the second formulation,

$$SA = \frac{6}{(1.170 \text{ } g/cm^3)(911\times10^{-4} cm)} = 56.29 \text{ cm}^2/g \text{ or } 56.29 \times 10^{-4} \text{ m}^2/g$$

PROBLEM 16.10.(a) From linear regression analysis we obtain

$$\frac{p}{x(p_o - p)} = 123.98 + (7096.56)\frac{p}{p_o}$$

The intercept is $I = \frac{1}{x_m b} = 123.98 \text{ g}^{-1}$.

The slope is $S = \frac{b - 1}{x_m b} = 7096.56 \text{ g}^{-1}$.

(b) From the BET equation, solving for x_m,

$$x_m = \frac{1}{S + I} = \frac{1}{7096.56 + 123.98} = 1.3849 \times 10^{-4} \text{ g/g}$$

$$V_m = \frac{x_m (g/g)}{\rho (g/cm^3)} = \frac{1.3849\times10^{-4} g/g}{1.25\times10^{-3} g/cm^3} = 0.110792 \text{ cm}^3/g$$

$$S_w = 4.35 \text{ m}^2/cm^3 \times 0.110792 \text{ cm}^3/g = 0.4819 \text{ meter}^2/g$$

$$d_{vs} = \frac{6}{\rho S_w} = \frac{6}{(1.455 \text{ } g/cm^3)(0.4819 \text{ } m^2/g)(10000 \text{ } cm^2)}$$

$$= 8.56 \times 10^{-4} \text{ cm} = 8.56 \text{ } \mu m$$

PROBLEM 16.11. S_w(before) $= 4.35 V_m = (4.35)(3.4) = 14.79 \text{ m}^2/g$
S_w(after) $= 4.35 V_m = (4.35)(260) = 1131 \text{ m}^2/g$

PROBLEM 16.12. See Figure P16 – 3.
From regression analysis, intercept, $I = 0.0120$; slope, $S = 0.260$;

$$V_m = \frac{1}{S + I} = \frac{1}{0.260 + 0.0120} = 3.676 \text{ cm}^3/g$$

$$S_w = (4.35 \text{ m}^2/cm^3)(3.676 \text{ cm}^3/g) = 15.99 \text{ m}^2/g \text{ or } 1.59 \times 10^5 \text{ cm}^2/g$$

$$d_{vs} = \frac{6}{\rho S_w} =$$

$$\frac{6}{(5.60 \ g/cm^3)(1.59 \times 10^5 \ cm^2/g)} =$$

6.7×10^{-6} cm $= 0.067 \ \mu m$

PROBLEM 16.13.

$$d_{vs} = \frac{(3.80)(2.19) \ cm}{[(1.267 \ cm^2)(2.19 \ cm) - 1]^{3/2}}$$

$$\times \sqrt{\frac{25 \ cm}{50 \ cm - 25 \ cm}};$$

$d_{vs} = 3.52 \times 10^{-4}$ cm

$$S_w = \frac{6}{(1.455 \ g/cm^3)(3.52 \times 10^{-4} \ cm)} = 1.17 \times 10^4 \ cm^2/g = 1.17 \ m^2/g$$

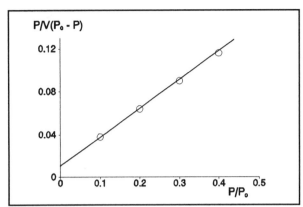

Figure P16-3 for Problem 16.12

The USP requires that the specific surface S_w for griseofulvin powder is not less than 1.3 m^2/g or more than 1.7 m^2/g. Therefore, the griseofulvin of this problem does not meet official specifications.

PROBLEM 16.14.

$$\ln p/p_o = -\frac{2(18.015)(72.8)}{(6.02 \times 10^{23})(1.381 \times 10^{-16})(0.998)(5.30 \times 10^{-7})(293.15)}$$

$= -0.2034; \ p/p_o = 0.816$

PROBLEM 16.15.(a) See Figure P16-4.

(b) From the Kelvin equation,

$r = -[2\gamma V/RT \ln(p/p_o)] =$

$$\frac{2(72.8)(18)}{(8.3143 \times 10^7)(293)\ln(p/p_o)}$$

At $p/p_o = 0.2$,

$r = 6.7 \times 10^{-8}$ cm

$= 6.7$ Å. The results are found in Table P16-3.

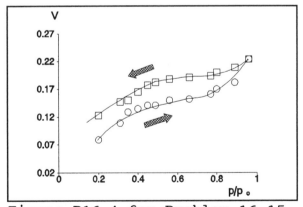

Figure P16-4 for Problem 16.15

Table P16 – 3 for Problem 16.15.

V_2 desorption (ml/g)	p/p_o	radius (Å)	Cum. pore vol.%
0.123	0.2	< 6.7	54.9
0.147	0.31	< 9.2	65.6
0.150	0.35	< 10.3	67
0.165	0.40	< 11.8	73.7
0.177	0.45	< 13.5	79.0
0.182	0.49	< 15.1	81.3
0.188	0.56	< 18.6	83.9
0.191	0.66	< 30	85.3
0.194	0.77	< 41.3	86.6
0.200	0.80	< 48.4	89.3
0.209	0.89	< 92.8	93.3
0.224	0.96	< 265	100

(c) The total pore volume is 0.224 ml/g corresponding to the intersection of both curves as read from Figure P16 – 4 and found in Table P16 – 3. It corresponds to a pore volume of 100%. Therefore, for, say, pores of radius < 92.8 Å, the cumulative pore volume in percentage is % = $\dfrac{0.209}{0.224}$ x 100 = 93.3%; the value 0.209 is ml/g taken from the desorption isotherm. The results are given in Table P16 – 3.

(d) From the Kelvin equation, these radii correspond to the following p/p_o values:

$$\ln (p/p_o) = -\frac{2\gamma V}{RTr} = -\frac{1.08 \times 10^{-7}}{40 \times 10^{-8}} = -0.270; \ p/p_o = 0.763$$

$$\ln (p/p_o) = -\frac{1.08 \times 10^{-7}}{60 \times 10^{-8}} = -0.18; \ p/p_o = 0.835$$

From the Figure P16 – 4 one can read the corresponding values for each p/p_o value (see also Table P16 – 3).

From the plot, for $p/p_o = 0.835$, $V_2 = 0.205$ ml/g and for $p/p_o = 0.763$, $V_2 = 0.193$ ml/g Therefore, since the volume of pores V_2 having radius, $r < 60$ Å is 0.205 and the volume of pores V_2 with radii < 40 Å is 0.193 ml/g, the volume of pores between $40 - 60$ Å is 0.205 $- 0.193 = 0.012$ ml/g. The total volume (100%) is 0.224, therefore $\% = \dfrac{0.012}{0.224} \times 100$ $= 5.5\%$ of pores with radius between $40 - 60$ Å.

PROBLEM 16.16. Apparent density $= \dfrac{75}{62} = 1.20967$;

$\%$ porosity $= \dfrac{4.0 - 1.20967}{4.0} \times 100 = 69.8\%$

PROBLEM 16.17.(a) Bulk density $= \dfrac{0.2626}{0.0836} = 3.14$ g/ml

(b) $\%$ porosity $= \dfrac{3.202 - 3.14}{3.202} \times 100 = 1.9\%$

PROBLEM 16.18. Bulk density $= \dfrac{324}{200} = 1.62$

$\%$ porosity $= \dfrac{2.70 - 1.62}{2.70} \times 100 = 40\%$

PROBLEM 16.19. $\%$ porosity $= \dfrac{1.37 - 1.33}{1.37} \times 100 = 3\%$

PROBLEM 16.20. $\%$ porosity $= \dfrac{3.203 - 3.138}{3.203} \times 100 = 2\%$

CHAPTER 17
Rheology

PROBLEM 17.1. (a). The equation is written in logarithmic form, (equation $17-6$)

$$\ln \eta = \ln A + E_v/RT$$

The energy of activation, E_v, and the value of $\ln A$ are obtained from the slope and intercept of a regression analysis of $\ln \eta$ against $1/T$. The data at different temperatures are shown in Table $P17-1$ and plotted in Figure $P17-1$. The equation is

$$\ln \eta = -6.30 + 1853.87 \frac{1}{T};$$

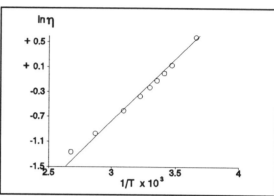

Figure P17-1 for Problem 17.1

slope $= 1853.87 = (E_v/R)$

$E_v = 1853.87 \times 1.9872 = 3684$ cal/mole

Intercept $= -6.30 = \ln A$; $A = \exp(-6.30) = 0.0018$

Table $P17-1$. Viscosity of water (CRC, 63rd ed., p. $F-40$). For Problem 17.1.

Temperature, °C	$1/T$ (x 10^3) °K^{-1}	η (cp)	$\ln \eta$
0	3.661	1.787	0.5805
15	3.470	1.139	0.1302
20	3.411	1.002	0.0020
25	3.354	0.8904	-0.11608
30	3.299	0.7975	-0.2263
37	3.224	0.6915	-0.3689
50	3.095	0.5468	-0.6037
75	2.872	0.3781	-0.9726
100	2.680	0.2818	-1.2666

(b) Using the linear regression equation, at T = 29°C(302.15°K), 1/T = 0.0033096,
ln η = − 6.30 + 1853.87(0.0033096) = − 0.16443; η = 0.8484 cp at 29°C.
Analogous calculations give η = 0.6231 cp at 45°C and η = 0.3114 cp at 88°C

$$\textbf{PROBLEM 17.2.} \quad U = \frac{K\,(w - w_f)}{v} = \frac{50\,(1800 - 1420)}{500} = 38 \text{ poise}$$

PROBLEM 17.3.(a) The calculated G and F values are given in Table P17 − 2. Figure
P17 − 2 shows a plot of G versus F, and Figure P17 − 3 shows a plot of ln G against ln F.
(b) The logarithmic expression, equation (17 − 9), is used together with the values found in
Table P17 − 2 for ln G and ln F, to obtain a linear least square fit of the data. The resulting
equation is ln G = N ln F − ln η' = 2.624 ln F − (11.578); r^2 = 0.9922
ln η' = +11.578; η' = 106,724 dyne sec/cm^2, and N = 2.624 (dimensionless)

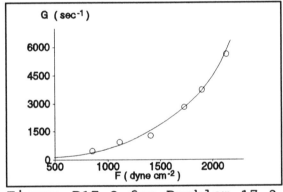

Figure P17-2 for Problem 17.3

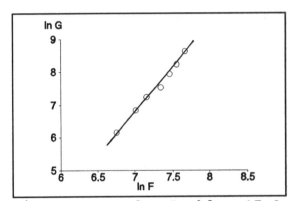

Figure P17-3 for Problem 17.3

Table P17 − 2 for Problem 17.3

G (sec^{-1}) = n×K$_G$	468.8	937.5	1406.3	1875.0	2812.5	3750.0	5625.0
F (dyne cm^{-2}) = S×K$_F$	853.6	1109.7	1280.4	1536.5	1728.5	1899.3	2134.0
ln G	6.150	6.843	7.249	7.536	7.942	8.230	8.635
ln F	6.749	7.012	7.155	7.337	7.455	7.549	7.666

(c) When the system is newtonian, N = 1 and as the system becomes non-newtonian N increases in value; in this case to N = 2.624.

(d) For G = 1875, ln G = 7.536

$$\ln F = \frac{\ln G + \ln \eta'}{N} = \frac{7.536 + 11.578}{2.624} = 7.2843; \quad F = 1457 \text{ dyne/cm}^2$$

PROBLEM 17.4. $U = \dfrac{F - f}{G};$

F − f = U G;

F = U G + f in which F = shearing stress, G = rate of shear and f = the yield value. Plotting F on the y−axis and G on the x−axis (Figure P17−4), the value of f is given by the y−intercept. Using regression analysis one obtains

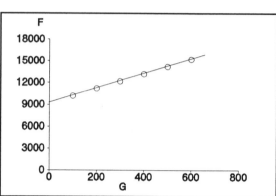

Figure P17-4 for Problem 17.4

F = 10.0 G + 9200. Thus U = 10.0 poise and f = 9200 dyne cm^{-2}

PROBLEM 17.5. Using equation (17 − 7),

$$U_1 = \frac{9440 - 5000}{240} = 18.5 \text{ poise}$$

$$U_2 = \frac{6728 - 5000}{240} = 7.20 \text{ poise}$$

Using equation (17 − 10),

$$B = \frac{U_1 - U_2}{\ln \dfrac{t_2}{t_1}} = \frac{18.5 - 7.20}{\ln \dfrac{80}{50}} = 24.04 \text{ dyne sec cm}^{-2}$$

PROBLEM 17.6. Using equation (7 − 23), $U = \dfrac{K_v (w - w_f)}{v}$ (see Example 17 − 7),

$$U_1 = \frac{(40.5)(269 - 124)}{543} = 10.8 \text{ poise or 11 poise}$$

$$U_2 = \frac{(40.5)(225 - 96)}{325} = 16.07 \text{ poise.}$$

From equation (17 − 24), $f = K_f w_f;$

$f_1 = (15.9)(124) = 1971.6$ dyne/cm^2;

$f_2 = (15.9)(96) = 1526$ dyne/cm^2

From equation (17 − 11),

$$M = \frac{(U_1 - U_2)}{\ln (v_2/v_1)} = \frac{(11 - 16)}{\ln (325/543)} \cong 10 \text{ dyne sec cm}^{-2}$$

PROBLEM 17.7. $K_v = \dfrac{\eta \, v}{w} = \dfrac{(200)(400)}{1600} = 50$ poise g^{-1} min^{-1}

PROBLEM 17.8. (See Figure P17 – 5). The slope is (rpm/mass) in the equation $K_v = \eta \times$ (rpm/mass). From linear regression analysis, intercept = a = 2.533 instead of zero as it should be.
Slope = b = 1.3317; r^2 = 0.9998.
K_v = 1.455 x 1.3317 = 1.9376 poise.
Using the instrumental constant K_v, the viscosity is calculated from:
$\eta = K_v$ (mass/rpm);
η = 1.9376(50/67.5) = 1.435 poise

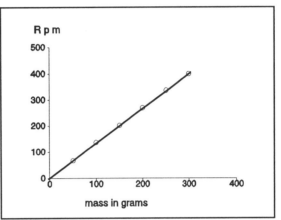

Figure P17-5 for Problem 17.8

Oil no. 1, $\eta = K_v$ (mass/rpm) = K_v (1/slope) = (1.9376)(1/0.216) = 8.970 poise (calibrated oil value = 9.344 poise).
Oil no. 6, η = (1.9376)(1/2.79) = 0.694 poise (calibrated oil value = 0.6725 poise)
Oil no. 9, η = (1.9376)(1/18.6) = 0.104 poise (calibrated oil value = 0.09134 poise)

PROBLEM 17.9. Figure P17-6 shows the plot of rpm against "weight". The more correct term is mass. Weight is actually mass x acceleration due to gravity; however the term weight is sometimes misused instead of mass as done in this problem. From equation (17 – 22),
$\eta = K_v$ (wt/rpm); rpm = (8.460/η) x wt.
Linear regression analysis of rpm against wt gives:
rpm = 0.142857 + 1.415357 (wt)
(r^2 = 0.9999)

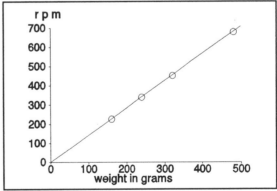

Figure P17-6 for Problem 17.9

The slope is 8.460/η = 1.415357 or 1/η
= slope/8.460 = (1.415357)/(8.460) = 0.1672999; η = 5.9773 poise or 597.7 cps
Note Slope = rpm/wt, not wt/rpm

PROBLEM 17.10. (a) Using equation (17 – 25),

$$\eta = C\frac{T}{v} = \frac{(1.168)(120)}{55} = 2.55 \text{ poise}$$

(b) From equation (17 – 26),

$$U = \frac{(T - T_f)}{v}C = \left(\frac{110 - 25}{200}\right)1.168 = 0.50 \text{ poise}$$

(c) From equation (17 – 27),

f = $C_f T_f$ = 0.122 x 25 = 3.1 dyne/cm^2

PROBLEM 17.11. For oil no. 1, $\eta = \frac{T}{v}C = \frac{169}{73.0} \times 1.168 = 2.704$ poise

For oil no. 2, $\eta = \frac{T}{v}C = \frac{95}{73.0} \times 1.168 = 1.520$ poise

For oil no. 3, $\eta = \frac{T}{v}C = \frac{49.4}{73.0} \times 1.168 = 0.7904$ poise

PROBLEM 17.12.(a) $C_f = \frac{3 \times 1923}{2\pi \times (2.007)^3} = 113.57 \text{ cm}^{-3}$

(b) f = 113.57 x 34.51 = 3919 dyne/cm^2

(c) $U = C\frac{T - T_f}{v} = 6.277\left(\frac{137.74 - 34.51}{73}\right) = 8.876 \text{ poise}$

PROBLEM 17.13. η (sample) = η (ref) $\frac{(\rho\ t)\ sample}{(\rho\ t)\ ref.}$

η (CS$_2$) = (1.002) $\frac{(1.2632)\ (85.1\ )}{(0.9982)\ (297.3\ )}$ = 0.363 cp. The CRC Handbook of Chemistry

and Physics, 63rd Ed., p. F – 42 gives η = 0.363 cp at 20°C

PROBLEM 17.14.

(a) η (olive oil) = 84.0 cp = 1.002 $\frac{(0.910)\ t\ (olive\ oil)}{(0.9982)\ (297.3)}$;

t (olive oil) = 27339 sec or 7.59 hours

We have chosen a pipette with too small a radius. Furthermore we should use a liquid of higher viscosity as the reference.

PROBLEM 17.15. Using Poiseuille's law, equation (17 − 13),

$\eta = \dfrac{\pi \, \Delta P \, r^4 \, t}{8 \, \ell \, V}$; and solving for ΔP,

ΔP = 8(0.04 dyne sec cm^{-2})(0.50 cm)(1.20 x 10^{-6} cm^3 sec^{-1})×
(7.5 x 10^{-4} mm Hg/dyne cm^{-2})/(π)(8.45 x 10^{-4} cm)^4 ; ΔP = 90 mm Hg;
1.01327 x 10^6 dyne cm^{-2} = 101,327 N m^{-2}; and 7.5 x 10^{-4} mm Hg = 1 dyne cm^{-2}. See
the front fly leaf in Physical Pharmacy for these physical constants.

90 mm Hg $\times \dfrac{1 dyne \; cm^{-2}}{7.5 \times 10^{-4} \; mm \; Hg} \times \dfrac{101,327 \; N \, m^{-2}}{1.01327 \times 10^6 \; dyne \; cm^{-2}}$ = 1.20 x 10^4 N m^{-2}

PROBLEM 17.16. $V/t = \dfrac{\pi \, \Delta P \, r^4}{8 \, \eta \, \ell}$

$= \dfrac{\pi \; (2.67 \times 10^4 \; dyne/cm^2) \; (0.0012 \; cm)^4}{(8 \times 0.04 \; dyne \; sec/cm^2 \times 0.32 \; cm)}$ = 1.70 x 10^{-6} cm^3/sec

PROBLEM 17.17. $\eta = \dfrac{\pi \; (\Delta P) \; r^4}{8 \; (V/t) \; \ell}$

$= \dfrac{\pi \; (6.93 \; dyne/cm^2) \times (0.5 \; cm)^4}{(8 \times 4.8 \; cm^3/sec \times 1 \; cm)}$ = 0.0354 dyne sec/cm^2

= 0.0354 poise = 3.54 cp

PROBLEM 17.18. A word statement problem. No calculations involved.

CHAPTER 18
Coarse Dispersions

PROBLEM 18.1. (a) The total surface area is $A = n\pi d^2$ where n is the number of particles and d the diameter.[a]

$A = (10^3)(3.1416)(10^{-3})^2 = 3.1416 \times 10^{-3}$ cm^2

The total surface energy is

$G = \gamma_{ls} A = (100)(3.1416 \times 10^{-3}) = 0.314$ erg

(b) The initial volume of a particle is $V = \frac{1}{6}\pi d^3 = \frac{1}{6}(3.1416)(10^{-3})^3 = 5.24 \times 10^{-10}$

cm^3. After dividing the solid particles, the volume of a new particle is

$V' = (5.24 \times 10^{-10})/100 = 5.234 \times 10^{-12}$ cm^3. Therefore the new diameter is

$d = \left(\frac{6\,V'}{\pi}\right)^{1/3} = \left(\frac{(6)\,(5.24 \times 10^{-12})}{3.1416}\right)^{1/3} = 2.15 \times 10^{-4}$ cm, and the new total surface

area is $A' = n'\pi d^2 = (10^3)(100)(3.1416)(2.15 \times 10^{-4})^2 = 0.0145$

The total surface free energy for the divided particles is:

$G' = (100)(0.0145) = 1.45$ erg

PROBLEM 18.2. $v = \dfrac{d^2\,(\rho - \rho_o)\,g}{18\,\eta_o}$

$= \dfrac{(100 \times 10^{-4})^2\,(2.44 - 1.01)\,981}{(18)\,(27)} = 2.9 \times 10^{-4}$ cm/sec

PROBLEM 18.3. $v = \dfrac{2}{9}\,\dfrac{r^2\,(\rho - \rho_o)\,g}{\eta}$

$= \dfrac{2\,(5 \times 10^{-5})^2\,(2.5 - 1.1)\,981}{(9)\,(5)} = 1.5 \times 10^{-7}$ cm/sec

PROBLEM 18.4.(a) n is computed from the slope of a plot of log v' against log ϵ. See Figure P18-1. The intercept gives the log of the velocity of sedimentation, v_{st}, found in Stokes' law. The data needed are given in Table P18-1. The regression line is:

---

[a] The student may use the value 3.1416 for π as done here or obtain π on the hand calculator to 9 decimal places which alters the answer slightly.

Table P18 – 1 for Problem 18.4.

log ε	-0.046	-0.022	-0.013	-0.004
log v'	-2.785	-1.420	-0.896	-0.382

log v' = 57.2284 log ε – 0.155
Slope = n = 57.2284 or 57.23;
intercept = log v_{st} = – 0.155;
v_{st} = 0.70 cm/sec
(b) The value obtained for v_{st} in part **(a)** is introduced in the Stokes equation to calculate the diameter of the particles:

$$d^2_{st} = \frac{v_s 18 \eta_o}{(\rho - \rho_o) g} =$$

$$\frac{(0.70)(18)(0.01)}{(3.15 - 1)981} = 5.97 \times 10^{-5};$$

$d_{st} = (5.97 \times 10^{-5})^{1/2} = 7.7 \times 10^{-3}$ cm = 77 μm

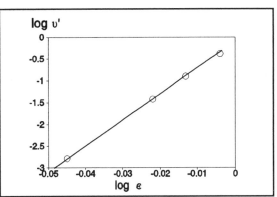

Figure P18-1 for Problem 18.4

PROBLEM 18.5. (Figure P18 – 2). Note that the horizontal axis is expressed using a logarithm scale. This makes it a little more difficult to interpret the ζ and H_u/H_o curves, but it is necessary because of the wide range of $AlCl_3$ concentrations. The caking region on the left is easily recognized and the concentration of $AlCl_3$ resulting in a hard cake falls between 0 and 1.0 mmole/liter. The noncaking region (see column 4 of Table 18 – 3 for a description of the caking conditions) is seen by the horizontal (maximum) plateau of the H_u/H_o values to fall between 1.0 mmole/liter and approximately 100 to 600 mmole/liter $AlCl_3$ concentration. Beyond 600 mmole/liter $AlCl_3$, the H_u/H_o curve drops off more sharply and the caking condition is expressed as a viscous mass, which probably forms a caked suspension over a period of time. Thus we have incipient caking on the left and right sides of Figure P18 – 2 and a noncaking region between. Unlike the case of the bismuth subnitrate cake in Figure P18 – 4, where KH_2PO_4 is the flocculating agent and tends to change the charge on bismuth subnitrate from positive to negative, the flocculating agent $AlCl_3$ in Figure P18 – 2 changes the charge from ordinarily negatively charged sulfamerazine to positive. The principle in the two cases is the same, with the formation of suspension caking and noncaking regions. When the ζ potential becomes relatively small, – 30 to +5 millivolts, flocculation and noncaking of the suspension occurs. At about 400 mmole/liter of $AlCl_3$, the ζ potential value reverts back from positive to negative; it is not clear at present why the latter occurs.

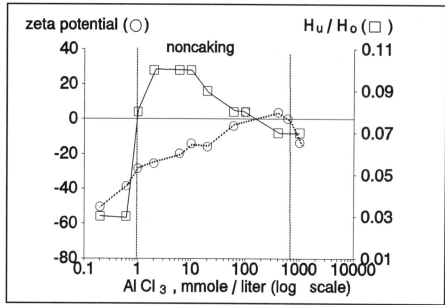

Figure P18-2 for Problem 18.5

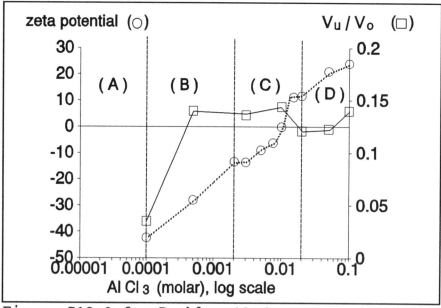

Figure P18-3 for Problem 18.6

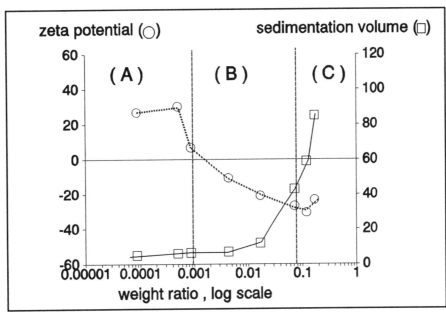

Figure P18-4 for Problem 18.7

PROBLEM 18.6. (Figure P18−3). The different zones are labeled as A, B, C and D. (A), caking region, (B), caked but easily dispersed, (C), noncaking and (D), ζ potential and possibility of caking increasing over time. As the charge increases due to the addition of AlCl$_3$ the system passes through the stages from caking to noncaking and returns to a possible caking condition.

PROBLEM 18.7. See Figure P18−4. The sedimentation volume increases with increasing bentonite/bismuth subnitrate ratios (mixtures 1−7 in Table 18−5), showing the largest rate of increase near mixture 5. At about this point, the zeta potential has the smallest absolute values and the sign changes from positive to negative. The smaller electrostatic repulsion allows the van der Waals forces to favor flocculation and to produce large sedimentation volumes.

Sedimentation volume continues to increase as bentonite concentrations increase in the region where the zeta potential drops to a relatively large negative value in Figure P18−4 (mixtures 7 and 13−16 in Table 18−5). Schott attributes this phenomenon to the formation of a thixotropic house−of−cards structure by the excess nonadsorbed bentonite, producing a viscous suspending medium.

PROBLEM 18.8. $V = \dfrac{4}{3}\pi r^3 = \dfrac{4}{3}(3.1416)(0.5 \times 10^{-4})^3$

$= 523.6 \times 10^{-15}$ cm^3/droplet.

The number of droplets per liter is $\dfrac{1000}{523.6 \times 10^{-15}}$ = 1.91 x 10^{15} particles;

The mole/liter of sodium oleate at the interface is 2 x 10^{-2}.

mole/droplet = $\dfrac{2 \times 10^{-2}\ mole/\ell}{1.91 \times 10^{15}\ droplet/\ell}$ = 1.0472 x 10^{-17}; molecules/droplet =

(1.0472 x 10^{-17} mole/droplet)(6.02 x 10^{23} molecule/mole) = 6.304 x 10^6 molecule/droplet.

Area per droplet = $4\pi r^2$ = (4)(3.1416)(0.5 x $10^{-4})^2$ = 314.16 x 10^{-10} cm^2

Area/molecule = $\dfrac{314.16 \times 10^{-10}}{6.304 \times 10^6}$ = 4.98 x 10^{-15} cm^2 = 50 Å^2.

PROBLEM 18.9. $\Delta G = \gamma \times \Delta A$ = (5 erg/cm^2) x 10^8 cm^2 = 5 x 10^8 erg;

$\dfrac{5 \times 10^8\ erg}{4.184 \times 10^7\ erg/cal}$ = 12 cal;   5 x 10^8 erg = 50 joule.

PROBLEM 18.10. Ratio Span/Tween = $\dfrac{40}{60}$;

% Span = $\dfrac{40}{100}$ x 100 = 40% ; % Tween = 60%.

HLB of mixture = (HLB$_1$ x fraction of 1 + HLB$_2$ x fraction of 2) = [(4.3)(0.4) + (15)(0.6)]
= 10.72

PROBLEM 18.11.(a) The RHLB for the oil phase of the w/o lotion is obtained by multiplying the fraction of each oil – phase ingredient by its RHLB and summing the values.

Table P18 – 2 for Problem 18.11.

	Amount	Fraction of oil phase	Individual RHLB's	
Mineral oil, light	10 g	0.18	11	= 1.98
Petrolatum	25 g	0.45	10	= 4.50
Stearic acid	15 g	0.27	17	= 4.59
Beeswax	5 g	0.09	9	= 0.81
$\sum$ = 55 g			RHLB of oil phase 11.88	

(b) The emulsifier consists of a combination of Arlacel 60 (HLB = 4.7) and Tween 60 (HLB = 14.9). To obtain the percentage of Arlacel and Tween in the 2 grams of emulsifier, the following equation is used

% (Hi HLB) = $\dfrac{RHLB - LoHLB}{HiHLB - LoHLB}$ x 100 , where "Hi" and "Lo" refer to the HLB of the surfactant of higher and lower HLB, respectively. Thus

% (Hi HLB) = $\dfrac{11.88 - 4.7}{14.9 - 4.7}$ x 100 = 70 %

The % of Tween 60 (the surfactant of higher HLB) is 70% of 2 grams or 1.4 g. The remainder, 0.6 g of Arlacel 60, is mixed with 1.4 g of Tween 60 to yield an oil in water emulsified lotion.

(c) The oil phase ingredients are heated together to a temperature of about 70°C. The water and the preservative phase is heated to about 73°C. Add the second to the first phase with mechanical stirring. When the product has nearly reached room temperature, add the perfume with continued stirring.

PROBLEM 18.12. (a) The data are listed in Table P18 – 3. The regression equation is

$\ln\left(\dfrac{M_t}{M_o}\right) = 0.700 \ln t + 0.224$

Intercept = ln k = 0.224; k = 1.251 % min$^{-0.7}$
From the slope, n = 0.7

The equation can be written as $\left(\dfrac{M_t}{M_o}\right) = 1.251\ t^{0.7}$

t > 0.5. It does not follow a Fickian model

(b) Fractional release, F % at 73 minutes is

$\ln\left(\dfrac{M_t}{M_o}\right)$ % = 0.700 ln(73 min) + 0.224 = 3.227; $\left(\dfrac{M_t}{M_o}\right)$ = 25.2 %

(c) ln t = [ln(100) − 0.224]/0.70 = 6.259; t = 522.6 min

Table P18 – 3 for Problem 18.12.

ln t	2.303	2.996	3.912	4.605	5.298
ln (M_t/M_o)	1.837	2.323	2.964	3.450	3.935

Table P18 – 4 for Problem 18.13.

t (hr)	0.5	1	1.5	2	3	4
t/W	0.176	0.251	0.326	0.401	0.551	0.701

PROBLEM 18.13. (a) The data needed for the plot (Fig. P18 – 5) are given in Table P18 – 4. The regression equation is $t/W = 0.101 + 0.150\ t$; $r^2 = 1.000$
Intercept = $A = 0.101$. Initial swelling rate = $1/A = 1/0.101 = 9.90$ g/hr
Slope = $B = 0.150$. Equilibrium swelling = $1/B = 1/0.150 = 6.67$ g solution/g gelatin
For gelatin – cetylpyridinium chloride at 4 hours, according to the equation, $t/W = 0.101 +$

$(0.150 \times 4) = 0.701$; $4\ hr/W = 0.701$; $W = \dfrac{4}{0.701} = 5.71$ (g solution)/(g gelatin)

For gelatin – dicloxacillin sodium, the equation is $t/W = 0.0310 + 0.110\ t$
At t = 4 hours, $t/W = 0.0310 + (0.110 \times 4) = 0.471$

$W = \dfrac{4}{0.471} = 8.49$ (g solution)/(g gelatin)

The W value for plain gelatin at t = 4 hr is
$t/W = 0.0755 + (4 \times 0.132) = 0.604$;

$W = \dfrac{4}{0.604} = 6.62$ (g solution)/(g gelatin)

(b) Percent decrease of W due
to gelatin – cetylpyridinium chloride

$= \dfrac{5.71 - 6.62}{6.62} \times 100 = -13.7\ \%$

(c) Percent of increase over W due
to dicloxacillin sodium

$= \dfrac{8.49 - 6.62}{6.62} \times 100 = 28.2\ \%$

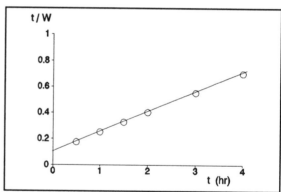

Figure P18-5 for Problem 18.13

PROBLEM 18.14. k_f and D_o can be computed from a regression of ln D against $\left(\dfrac{1}{H} - 1\right)$ according to the equation

$\ln D = \ln D_o - k_f\left(\dfrac{1}{H} - 1\right)$. The data needed are presented in Table P18 – 5.

Table P18 − 5 for Problem 18.14

$\left(\dfrac{1}{H} - 1\right)$	1.841	1.653	0.565	0.136
ln D	− 17.504	− 17.145	− 14.623	− 13.486

The equation is

$$\ln D = -13.223 - 2.354\left(\frac{1}{H} - 1\right); \; r = -0.999$$

$k_f = (-\text{slope}) = 2.354$ and the intercept is $\ln D_o = -13.223$; $D_o = 1.81 \times 10^{-6}$ cm^2/sec

PROBLEM 18.15. The regression equation is

$$\ln k = 20.202 - 9027.4\frac{1}{T}; \; r^2 = 0.9999$$

slope $= E_a/R$; $E_a = 9027.4 \times 1.9872 = 17{,}939$ cal/mole
The exponential equation is k (g^{-1} hr^{-1}) $= (5.938 \times 10^8)\, e^{-17939/RT}$

PROBLEM 18.16. (a) Regression of concentration remaining [A] against time, gives the following equations:
Brand B: $[A] = 300 - 7.758\, t$; $\quad r = -0.9999$
Brand E: $[A] = 300 - 2.815\, t \quad r = -1.000$
From the slopes, $k_o = 7.758$ (mg/5 ml)/day (Brand B)
$\qquad\qquad k_o = 2.815$ (mg/5 ml)/day (Brand E)
The initial concentration $[A_o] = 300$ mg/5 ml for both brands B and E is obtained from the intercepts on the y − axis.

(b) $\quad t_{90} = \dfrac{10\,\% \; decomposition \times A_o}{k_o}$; $k_o = \dfrac{(0 - 10)\,[A_o]}{t_{90}}$ for zero order kinetics,

Chapter 12, $\quad t_{90} = \dfrac{0.10\,[A]_o}{k_o} = \dfrac{0.10\,(300)}{7.758} = 3.9$ days (brand B) at 5°C

$t_{90} = \dfrac{0.10\,(300)}{2.815} = 10.6$ days (brand E) at 5°C. Product E meets the label requirements.

PROBLEM 18.17. The data needed are shown in Table P18 − 6
For acid catalysis:

$$\ln k_{H^+} = -11172.9\frac{1}{T} + 38.669; \; E_a = (11172.9)(1.9872) = 22{,}203 \text{ cal/mole}$$

Table P18 – 6 for Problem 18.17.

T (°C)	80°	50°	40°	23°
$1/T$ (°K^{-1}) x 10^3	2.833	3.096	3.195	3.378
ln k_{H^+}	6.632	4.284	3.800	0.278
ln k_{OH^-}	5.124	2.833	2.610	−0.989
ln k_o	−2.017	−4.457	−7.143	−6.751

For basic catalysis:

ln k_{OH^-} = $-10648.6 \frac{1}{T}$ + 35.667; E_a = (10648.6)(1.9872) = 21,161 cal/mole

For catalysis by the solvent

ln k_o = $-9545.1 \frac{1}{T}$ + 24.741; E_a = (9545.1)(1.9872) = 18,968 cal/mole

PROBLEM 18.18. The data needed for the plot are shown in Table P18 – 7:

Using regression analysis, one obtains:

$Q = 1.02 \times 10^{-3}$ mg/(cm^2 hr$^{1/2}$) $t^{1/2}$ (hr$^{1/2}$) + (6.1×10^{-6}) mg/cm^2

The intercept is practically zero

slope = release rate

= 1.02×10^{-3} mg cm^{-2} hr$^{-1/2}$

According to the Higuchi equation,

$Q = [D(2A - C_s)C_s]^{1/2}t^{1/2}$

slope = $\sqrt{D(2A - C_s)C_s}$

= 1.02×10^{-3} mg cm^{-2} hr$^{-1/2}$

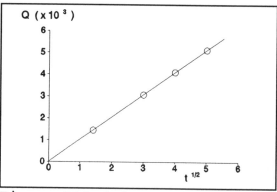

Figure P18-6 for Problem 18.18

Table P18 – 7 for Problem 18.18.

$t^{1/2}$ (hr$^{1/2}$)	1.41	3	4	5
$Q \times 10^3$ (mg/cm^2)	1.45	3.07	4.10	5.12

$D(2A - C_s)C_s = (1.02 \times 10^{-3})^2 = 1.04 \times 10^{-6} \text{ mg}^2 \text{ cm}^{-4} \text{ hr}^{-1}$

$D[(2 \times 20) - 2.121](2.121) = 1.04 \times 10^{-6}$

$D = 1.3 \times 10^{-8} \text{ cm}^2/\text{hr or } 3.6 \times 10^{-12} \text{ cm}^2/\text{sec}$

PROBLEM 18.19. For the release in μg from unit area, cm^2, of a suspension – ointment,

$Q = [D(2A - C_s)C_s]^{1/2}t^{1/2}$

For particle size = 88 μm, and after 9 hours the drug released is

$Q = [1.11 \times 10^{-6}(1200 - 495)495 \times 32,400 \text{ sec}]^{1/2} = 112 \ \mu g/\text{cm}^2$

For particle size = 5.1 μm, and after 9 hours the drug released is

$Q = [1.85 \times 10^{-6}(1200 - 495)495 \times 32,400 \text{ sec}]^{1/2} = 145 \ \mu g/\text{cm}^2$

Note that Q in μg drug release per unit area of ointment base is larger when the particle size is reduced.

PROBLEM 18.20. (a) If the cross – section area of soap molecule is 25 Å
= 25 x 10^{-16} cm^2 and the diameter of the oil globule is 1 μm, the surface area is

(surface area)/globule = $\pi d^2 = 3.1416 \times (1 \times 10^{-4} \text{ cm})^2 = 3.1416 \times 10^{-8} \text{ cm}^2$

(b) $\dfrac{3.1416 \times (1 \times 10^{-4})^2 \ cm^2/oil \ globule}{25 \times 10^{-16} \ cm^2 \ area/soap \ molecule} = 1.26 \times 10^7 = 12,600,000$ or 12.6 million

molecules of soap around each oil globule.

(c) The volume of each globule is $v = \dfrac{\pi d^3}{6} = \dfrac{\pi \times (10^{-4})^3}{6}$

$= 5.24 \times 10^{-13} \text{ cm}^3/\text{particle.}$

$\dfrac{50 \ cm^3 \ oil}{5.24 \times 10^{-13} \ cm^3/particle} = 9.5 \times 10^{13}$ particles of oil $\approx 10 \times 10^{13}$ particles or 100

trillion droplets of oil.

(d) 1.26 x 10^7 soap molecules/globule x (100 x 10^{12}) globules = 1.26 x 10^{21} soap molecules in our 100 cm^3 emulsion.

(e) The molecular weight of sodium stearate is approximately 300 g/mole.

$\dfrac{300 \ g/mole}{6.02 \times 10^{23} \ molecules/mole} = 50 \times 10^{-23}$ g of soap/molecule

(f) From the results **(d)** and **(e)**,

1.26 x 10^{21} soap molecules x (50 x 10^{-23}) g/soap molecule = 0.60 grams soap needed for the 100 cm^3 of emulsion to cover the 50 cm^3 of oil globules with a layer of soap one molecule thick.

(g) We finally arrived at the result 0.6 g of soap is needed. Ordinarily 1 or 2 grams of soap are used for such emulsions. If the oil particles are larger we will need less amount of soap because the total surface area of the oil globules is smaller.

PROBLEM 18.21. No calculations are required for this problem.

CHAPTER 19
Drug Product Design

PROBLEM 19.1. (a) $VW_3 = \frac{4}{3}\pi R^3 - VL_3 = \frac{4}{3}\pi(0.0447)^3 - 15.2 \times 10^{-5}$

$= 2.22 \times 10^{-4}\ \mu m^3$

(b) $TLV_3 = N_3 \times VL_3 = (52.7 \times 10^{14})(15.2 \times 10^{-5}) = 8.01 \times 10^{11}\ \mu m^3$

(c) $E = \dfrac{\frac{4}{3}\pi N R^3}{TLV} - 1 = \dfrac{\frac{4}{3}\pi(52.7 \times 10^{14})(0.0447)^3}{8.01 \times 10^{11}} - 1 = 1.46$

(d) $TSA_3 = 4\pi N_3 R_3{}^2 = 4\pi(52.7 \times 10^{14})(0.0447)^2) = 1.32 \times 10^{14}\ \mu m^2$

PROBLEM 19.2. (a) For the 3rd bilayer $R_3 = R_1 - [(3-1)(45.7\ \text{Å} + 60\ \text{Å})]$
where $R_1 = 5000\ \text{Å}$; $R_3 = 4788.6\ \text{Å}$
Analogous calculations give $R_2 = 4894.3\ \text{Å}$; $R_4 = 4682.9\ \text{Å}$ and $R_5 = 4577.2\ \text{Å}$

(b) $PE = \dfrac{(5000)^2}{(5000 + 4894 + 4789 + 4683 + 4577)^2} \times 100 = 4.36\%$

(c) $R_5' = 5000\ \text{Å} - [(45.7 \times 5) + 60(5 - 1)] = 4532\ \text{Å}$

$V_5' = \frac{4}{3}\pi(4532)^3 = 3.90 \times 10^{11}\ \text{Å}^3 = 0.39\ \mu m^3$

PROBLEM 19.3. (a) Volume $= \frac{1}{6}\pi(340 \times 10^{-4})^3\ cm^3 = 2.058 \times 10^{-5}\ cm^3$

(b) Mass $= 1.15\ g/cm^3 \times 2.058 \times 10^{-5}\ cm^3 = 2.37 \times 10^{-5}\ g$
or $2.37 \times 10^{-5}\ g \times 1\ \mu g/(10^{-6}\ g) = 23.67\ \mu g$

(c) $23.67\ \mu g \times 0.225 = 5.33\ \mu g$ in 0.5 ml or $10.66\ \mu g/ml$

PROBLEM 19.4. $\ln M = (\ln[\eta] - \ln K)/a = \dfrac{2.8622 + 6.3830}{0.950} = 9.7318$

$M = \exp(9.7318) = e^{9.7318} = 16{,}845$ daltons

PROBLEM 19.5.

$M = \dfrac{(0.80\ cm^2)(9.2 \times 10^{-9}\ cm^2/\sec)(1.83)(8\ mg/cm^3)}{0.01\ cm} \times (24\ hr \times 3600\ sec/hr)$

$= 0.931$ mg

Table P19 – 1 for Problem 19.6.

pH	4.67	5.67	6.24	6.40
P $(\times 10^6)$ cm/sec	4.885	5.280	6.169	6.564
J $(\times 10^{10})$ mole/(cm^2 sec)	1.80	1.95	2.27	2.42

PROBLEM 19.6. (a)   The ionized fraction, f_{BH^+}, for each pH value is

$f_{BH^+} = (1 - f_B)$. At pH 4.67,

$P = P_B f_B + P_{BH^+} f_{BH^+} = [(9.733 \times 10^{-6})(0.01)] + [(4.836 \times 10^{-6})(1 - 0.01)] = 4.885 \times 10^{-6}$ cm/sec. Similar calculations give P values at the several pH's (Table P19 – 1).

The total flux is $J = J_B + J_{BH^+} = (P_B f_B C_d) + (P_{BH^+} f_{BH^+} C_d) = C_d (P_B f_B + P_{BH^+} f_{BH^+}) = PC_d$

At pH 4.67, $J = (4.885 \times 10^{-6})(3.69 \times 10^{-5}) = 1.80 \times 10^{-10}$ mole/(cm^2 sec)

Calculations at this and the other pH's using the values of P found in Table P19 – 1 (2nd row), give the flux, J. (Table P19 – 1, 3rd row).

(b) Since $\dfrac{M}{S t} \cong J$, the total amount of penetrant at time t is M = J S t.

At pH 6.40 and 30 min,

$M = (2.42 \times 10^{-10})(0.95)(30 \times 60) = 4.13 \times 10^{-7}$ moles

The undissociated mass of penetrant M_B is

$M_B \cong S J_B t$ where

$J_B = P_B f_B C_d = 9.733 \times 10^{-6} \times 0.35 \times 3.69 \times 10^{-5} = 1.257 \times 10^{-10}$ mole/(cm^2 sec)

$M_B = 0.95 \times 1.257 \times 10^{-10} \times (30 \times 60) = 2.149 \times 10^{-7}$ moles

The dissociated form, $M_{BH^+} = S J_{BH^+} t$

$J_{BH^+} = P_{BH^+} f_{BH^+} C_d = 4.836 \times 10^{-6} (1 - 0.35)(3.69 \times 10^{-5})$

$= 1.160 \times 10^{-10}$ mole/cm^2 sec

$M_{BH^+} = (0.95)(1.160 \times 10^{-10})(30 \times 60) = 1.98 \times 10^{-7}$ mole

Another way to calculate M_{BH^+}:

$M_{BH^+} = M - M_B = (4.13 \times 10^{-7} - 2.149 \times 10^{-7}) = 1.98 \times 10^{-7}$ moles at t = 30 min.

Followig these steps, M_B and M_{BH^+} are calculated at t = 60 and t = 150 min (Table P19 – 2).

(c) The lag time is

$t_L = \dfrac{h}{6 P} = \dfrac{0.022 \; cm}{(6)(4.72 \times 10^{-6}) \; cm/sec} = 776.8$ sec ≈ 13 min

Table P19 – 2 for Problem 19.6.

t (min)	60	150
$M_B \times 10^7$ moles	4.30	10.75
$M_{BH^+} \times 10^7$ moles	3.97	9.94
M total x 10^7 moles	8.27	20.69

PROBLEM 19.7. (a) At low pH (pH = 2.4),
$[H^+] = 3.98 \times 10^{-3}$, $k_{obs} = 9.60 \times 10^{-3}$ min^{-1}

$$k_{HA} = \frac{k_{obs}}{\left(\frac{[H]^+}{[H]^+ + K_a}\right)} = \frac{9.60 \times 10^{-3}}{\left(\frac{3.98 \times 10^{-3}}{(3.98 \times 10^{-3}) + (6.30 \times 10^{-5})}\right)} = 9.75 \times 10^{-3} \text{ min}^{-1}$$

At high pH (pH 7.19), $[H^+] = 6.457 \times 10^{-8}$ and $k_{obs} = 2.40 \times 10^{-3}$ min^{-1}

$$k_{A^-} = \frac{k_{obs}}{\left(\frac{K_a}{[H]^+ + K_a}\right)} = \frac{2.40 \times 10^{-3}}{\left(\frac{6.30 \times 10^{-5}}{(6.457 \times 10^{-8}) + (6.30 \times 10^{-5})}\right)} = 2.40 \times 10^{-3} \text{ min}^{-1}$$

(b) At low pH (pH = 3), $[H^+] = 1.0 \times 10^{-3}$

$$k_{obs} = k_{HA}\left(\frac{[H]^+}{[H]^+ + K_a}\right) = (9.75 \times 10^{-3}) \times \left(\frac{1 \times 10^{-3}}{(1 \times 10^{-3}) + (6.30 \times 10^{-5})}\right)$$

$$= 9.17 \times 10^{-3} \text{ min}^{-1}$$

At high pH (pH = 8.2), $[H^+] = 6.310 \times 10^{-9}$

$$k_{obs} = k_{A^-}\left(\frac{K_a}{[H]^+ + K_a}\right) = 2.40 \times 10^{-3} \times \left(\frac{6.30 \times 10^{-5}}{(6.310 \times 10^{-9}) + (6.30 \times 10^{-5})}\right)$$

$$= 2.40 \times 10^{-3} \text{ min}^{-1}$$

PROBLEM 19.8. (a) See Figure P19 – 1. A regression of 1/V against 1/S gives the following equation:

1/V = 3008 + 1.428 1/S; r^2 = 0.971

$1/V_m$ = intercept = 3008; V_m = 3.324 x 10^{-4} hr^{-1}

(b) From the equation obtained in **(a)**,

slope $= K_m/V_m = 1.428$;

$K_m = (1.428)(3.324 \times 10^{-4})$

$= 4.75 \times 10^{-4}$ M

(c) The data are plotted in Figure P19–1. From the plot, the value of K_m is 4.75×10^{-4} M.

(d) $\dfrac{1}{V_m} = 3008 + 1.428\,\dfrac{1}{S}$

$= 3008 + 1.428(2347) = 6359.5$ M^{-1}hr;

$V = 1.57 \times 10^{-4}$ mole/(liter hr)

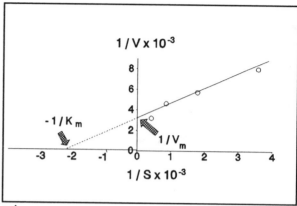

Figure P19-1 for Problem 19.8

PROBLEM 19.9. $B_{20} = \dfrac{A}{20\,RF}\left[n - \dfrac{\left(1 - e^{-\frac{nk}{RF}}\right)e^{-\frac{k}{RF}}}{1 - e^{-\frac{k}{RF}}}\right] =$

$\dfrac{30}{20 \times 14}\left[(20 \times 14) - \dfrac{\left(1 - e^{-\frac{(20 \times 14)0.058}{14}}\right)e^{\frac{-0.058}{14}}}{1 - e^{\frac{-0.058}{14}}}\right] = 12.3\ \mu g$

PROBLEM 19.10. The transferred amount at t = 40 min is computed from equation (19 – 23). As the first step, the transfer in 20 min is obtained, using equation (19 – 22):

$B_{20} = \dfrac{7.8}{20 \times 14}\left[(20 \times 14) - \dfrac{\left(1 - e^{-\frac{(20 \times 14)0.07}{14}}\right)e^{\frac{-0.07}{14}}}{1 - e^{\frac{-0.07}{14}}}\right] = 3.61\ \mu g$

wher B_{20} stands for the value of B at 20 minutes.

Then A_{20} is computed from equation (19 – 24).

$A_{20} = \left[\left(\dfrac{7.8}{20 \times 14}\right)(1 - e^{-20 \times 0.07})e^{\frac{-0.07}{14}}\right]\left(1 - e^{\frac{-0.07}{14}}\right) = 0.0001\ \mu g$

Finally, from equation (19 – 23) one obtains the value of B at t = 40 min:

$B_{40} = 3.61 + 0.0001[1 - e^{-0.07(40 - 20)}] = 3.61369 \cong 3.61\ \mu g$. B_{40} does not differ from B_{20} in the first 2 digits after the decimal point.

Table P19 − 3 for Problem 19.11

pH	0	1	2	3	4	5	6	7
(dM/dt) (g/sec)	0.00308	0.00321	0.0042	0.0147	0.119	1.163	11.60	116

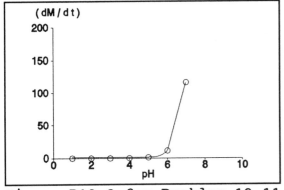
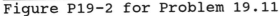

Figure P19-2 for Problem 19.11

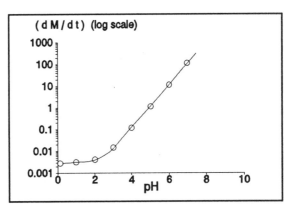

Figure P19-3 for Problem 19.11

PROBLEM 19.11. $\dfrac{dM}{dt} = \dfrac{DS}{h}\left(C_s\left(1 + \dfrac{K_a}{[H^+]}\right) - C_g\right)$; At pH 1, $[H^+] = 0.1$

$$\frac{dM}{dt} = \frac{(6.8 \times 10^{-7})\,(1.5 \times 10^4)}{8 \times 10^{-3}}\left[(2.6 \times 10^{-3})\left(1 + \frac{3.5 \times 10^{-3}}{0.1}\right) - 1.7 \times 10^{-4}\right]$$

= 0.00321 g/sec = 3.21 mg/sec. The calculated values of (dM/dt) at the various pH's are showm in Table P19 − 3. See additional problems like 19.11 in J. T. Carstensen, <u>Pharmaceutics of Solids and Solid Dosage Forms</u>, Wiley, New York, 1977, Chap. 13. Figure P19 − 2 shows a plot of (dM/dt) against pH. There is a sharp increase in the dissolution rate at pH 6. The rectangular plot does not differentiate the values of (dM/dt) from 0.00321 to 0.119 g/sec because the scale range is wide. To better show the variation of (dM/dt), a semilog plot of log (dM/dt) against pH is constructed. (Figure P19 − 3).

PROBLEM 19.12.

$$(dM/dt)_z = \frac{(2.0 \ cm^2)\,(120 \ atm)\,(5 \times 10^{-6} \ cm^2/atm \ hr)\,(750 \ mg/cm^3)}{0.019 \ cm} = 47.4 \text{ mg/hr}$$

PROBLEM 19.13. (a) Polymer dissolution rate, $v = S J$, where J is given by equation (19 − 41). At gastric pH:

$$v = 2\text{ cm}^2 \frac{(5 \times 10^{-8}\ cm^2/sec)\ (60\ sec/min)}{(50\ \mu m)\ (10^{-4}\ cm/\mu m)} (6\text{ mg/ml})\left(1 + \frac{10^{-4.5}}{10^{-1.5}}\right)$$

$$= 72 \times 10^{-4}\text{ mg/min}$$

Amount of coating required to dissolve before coating ruptures under gastric conditions = 90% of 10% of 400 mg = 36 mg

$$\text{Time required} = \frac{36\ mg}{72 \times 10^{-4}\ mg/min} = 5{,}000\text{ min} \approx 83\text{ hr in the gastric medium.}$$

Polymer dissolution rate at the intestinal conditions:

$$v = 2\text{ cm}^2 \frac{(5 \times 10^{-8}\ cm^2/sec)\ (60\ sec/min)}{(50\ \mu m)\ (10^{-4}\ cm/\mu m)} (6\text{ mg/ml})\left(1 + \frac{10^{-4.5}}{10^{-6.8}}\right) = 1.44\text{ mg/min}$$

$$\text{Time required for onset of disintegration} = \frac{36\ mg}{1.44\ mg/min} = 25\text{ min in the intestinal}$$

medium.

(b) Release meets specifications in the gastric and intestinal medium. If not, a slightly lower coating loading could be used, or an enteric coating polymer with lower pK_a and/or higher solubility.

PROBLEM 19.14. (a) The concentrations of $[H^+]$ and $[OH^-]$ in the bulk phase are:
$[H^+] = -\log pH = 1 \times 10^{-3}$; $[OH^-] = K_w/[H^+]_b = 10^{(-14 + 3)} = 1 \times 10^{-11}$
To make the calculations, involving the many terms in dissolution theory, diffusivity ratios for all ions in solution, OH^-, H^+, and BH^+ are defined:

$$\gamma_1 = \frac{D_{OH^-}}{D_{H^+}} = \frac{2.7 \times 10^{-5}}{2.7 \times 10^{-5}} = 1$$

$$\gamma_2 = \frac{D_{BH^+}}{D_{H^+}} = \frac{6.8 \times 10^{-6}}{2.7 \times 10^{-5}} = 0.25$$

The constants a, b and c (Table 19 – 1) are calculated as follows:
$a = K_a + \gamma_2[B]_o = (1.26 \times 10^{-6}) + (0.25 \times 3.08 \times 10^{-5}) = 8.96 \times 10^{-6}$ M
$b = (-[H^+] + \gamma_1[OH^-] - \gamma_2[BH^+])K_a$
$= [(-1 \times 10^{-3}) + (1 \times 10^{-11}) - (0.25 \times 0)](1.26 \times 10^{-6}) = -1.26 \times 10^{-9}$ M²
$c = \gamma_1 K_w K_a = 1 \times (1 \times 10^{-14})(1.26 \times 10^{-6}) = 1.26 \times 10^{-20}$ M²
The hydrogen ion concentration at the surface is:

$$[H^+]_s = \frac{-b + \sqrt{b^2 - 4ac}}{2a}$$

$$= \frac{+1.26 \times 10^{-9} + \sqrt{1.588 \times 10^{-18} + 4\ (8.96 \times 10^{-6})\ (1.26 \times 10^{-20})}}{(2)\ (8.96 \times 10^{-6})}$$

$= 1.406 \times 10^{-4}$ M ; $(pH)_s = 3.85$

The total concentration at the surface of the matrix, equation (19 – 43), is:

$$C_{T,s} = [B]_o\left(1 + \frac{[H^+]_s}{K_a}\right) = (3.08 \times 10^{-5})\left(1 + \frac{1.406 \times 10^{-4}}{1.26 \times 10^{-6}}\right) = 3.47 \times 10^{-3} \text{ M}$$

(b) From equation (19 – 41):

$$v = S\left[\frac{D_B}{h}(C_{T,s} - C_{T,b})\right] = 1.8 \text{ cm}^2 \frac{6.8 \times 10^{-6} \text{ cm}^2/\text{sec}}{0.01 \text{ cm}} (3.47 \times 10^{-3}) \text{ mole/cm}^3$$

$= 4.25 \times 10^{-6}$ mole cm^{-2} sec^{-1}.   Note: $c_{T,b} = 0$.

PROBLEM 19.15. Taking the antilog of both sides of equation (19 – 96),

$\dfrac{S_o}{S - S_o} = 10^{pH - pKa}$. Then inverting terms $\dfrac{S - S_o}{S_o} = \dfrac{1}{10^{pH - pK_a}}$;

$$S = \frac{S_o\left[1 + 10^{(pH - pK_a)}\right]}{10^{(pH - pK_a)}}$$

At pH 5.48,

$$S = \frac{0.0099\left[1 + 10^{(5.48 - 8.99)}\right]}{10^{(5.48 - 8.99)}} = 32 \text{ mg/ml}$$

Analogously, at pH 7.04,

$$S = \frac{0.0099\left[1 + 10^{(7.04 - 8.99)}\right]}{10^{(7.04 - 8.99)}} = 0.89 \text{ mg/ml}$$

PROBLEM 19.16 (a). The intrinsic carrier permeability, equation (19 – 35) is

$$P_c^{\star} = \frac{J_{max}^{\star}}{K_m} = \frac{9.1}{7.2} = 1.264$$

(b) The intrinsic wall permeability, equation (19 – 36) is

$$P_w^{\star} = \frac{P_c^{\star}}{1 + (c_w/K_m)} + P_m^{\star}$$

For $c_w = 0.01$ mM and $P_m^{\star} = 0$,

$$P_w^{\star} = \frac{1.264}{1 + (0.01/7.2)} = 1.262$$

Analogous calculations for the other concentration values give the results presented in Table P19 – 4.

Table P19−4 for Problem 19.16.

c_w (mM)	0.01	0.05	0.10	1.0	5.00	10.0	50.0	100
ln c_w	−4.605	−2.996	−2.303	0.000	1.609	2.303	3.912	4.6105
$P_w^\star$	1.262	1.255	1.247	1.110	0.746	0.529	0.159	0.085

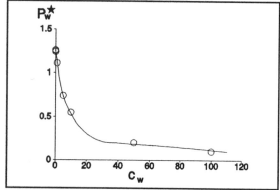

Figure 19-4 for Problem 19.16

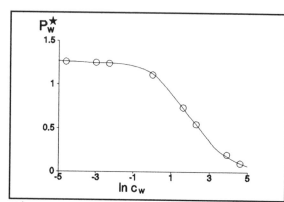

Figure 19-5 for Problem 19.16

(c) See Figures P19−4 and P19−5. As observed in Figure P19−5, a logarithmic relationhip in c_w does not yield a straight line. There is a inflection of the curve toward higher ln c_w values. See the paper by P. J. Sinko and G. L. Amidon, Pham. Res., **5**, 645, 1988 for more detail.

PROBLEM 19.17.(a) $\quad P_c^\star = \dfrac{J_{max}^\star}{K_m} = \dfrac{1.6}{1.5} = 1.067$

(b) $P_w^\star = \dfrac{P_c^\star}{1 + (c_w/K_m)} + P_m^\star;\quad$ for $c_w = 0.1, 7.2,$ and 50 mM

$P_w^\star = \dfrac{1.067}{1 + (0.10/1.50)} + 0.3 = 1.300;$

$P_w^\star = \dfrac{1.067}{1 + (7.2/1.50)} + 0.3 = 0.484;$

$P_w^\star = \dfrac{1.067}{1 + (50/1.50)} + 0.3 = 0.331$

Table P19 − 5 for Problem 19.18.

$P_w^\star$	0.5	1	1.5	2	2.5	3
F	0.609	0.847	0.940	0.977	0.991	0.996

PROBLEM 19.18.

(a) $G_z = \dfrac{\pi DL}{2 v_m} = \dfrac{(3.1416)(5.0 \times 10^{-6}\ cm^2/sec)(500\ cm)}{(2)(0.5/60\ cm^3/sec)} = 0.47$ (dimensionless).

(b) $F = 1 - e^{-4 G_z P_w^\star}$

For $P_w^\star = 0.5$, $F = 1 - e^{-4(0.47)(0.5)} = 0.609$

The results are presented in Table P19 − 5.

PROBLEM 19.19.
$V_{app} = K_{app}/(\text{body weight})^{0.75} = \dfrac{0.173\ min^{-1}}{(248\ g)^{0.75}}$

$= 0.00277\ min^{-1}\ g^{-1}$

$V_{app} = \dfrac{V_o + V_{-1}(K_a/[H^+])}{1 + K_a/[H^+]} = 0.00277\ min^{-1} g^{-1}$. Solve for $[H^+]$:

$0.00277\left(1 + \dfrac{1.74 \times 10^{-3}}{[H^+]}\right) = 57.312 \times 10^{-3} + 1.860 \times 10^{-3}\left(\dfrac{1.74 \times 10^{-3}}{[H^+]}\right)$

Rearranging terms,

$0.00277 - (57.312 \times 10^{-3}) = \dfrac{3.236 \times 10^{-6} - 4.820 \times 10^{-6}}{[H^+]};$

$[H^+] = 2.90 \times 10^{-5};\quad pH = 4.54$

PROBLEM 19.20.
$\pi = \dfrac{2(100\ g/\ell)(0.082\ \ell\ atm/mole\ degree)(310\ degree)}{254.2\ g/mole} = 20\ atm$

PROBLEM 19.21.
$S_{max} = \dfrac{10 \times 10^{-4}\ cm}{50}(35\ mg/hr)\dfrac{1}{(0.0226\ cm^2/hr)(750\ mg/cm^3)}$

$S_{max} = 4.13 \times 10^{-5}\ cm^2 = 4130\ \mu m^2$
(Note: $1\ cm = 10^4\ \mu m$ so $1\ cm^2 = 10^4 \times 10^4 = 10^8\ \mu m^2$)
This area, $S_{max} = \pi\ r^2$; $4130\ \mu m^2 = 3.1416\ r^2$;

r = 36.3 μm and diameter = 72.5 μm

PROBLEM 19.22. From equation (19 – 59),

$$\lambda = \frac{(8)\,(6.915\times10^{-3}\ poise)\,(3.24\times10^{-5}\ cm^2/sec)}{(8.3143\times10^{7}\ erg\,°K^{-1}mole^{-1})\,(310\ °K)\,/\,(18.14\ cm^2/mole)} \times$$

(17.48 – 1) = 2.08 x 10^{-14} cm

From equation (19 – 58),

r = – 1.5 x 10^{-8} cm + (2 x 2.25 x 10^{-16} cm^2 + 2.08 x $10^{-14})^{1/2}$
= 13.1 x 10^{-8} cm = 13.1 Å

PROBLEM 19.23. (a) The concentration of ionized species at pH 7 is

$$[A^-] = \frac{10^{(pH\,-\,pK_a)}}{1\,+\,10^{(pH\,-\,pK_a)}}[T] = \frac{10^{(7\,-\,4.5)}}{1\,+\,10^{(7\,-\,4.5)}} \times 916.6 = 913.71\ \mu g/ml$$

The concentration of nonionized species is [HA] = [T] – [A$^-$]
= 916.6 – 913.71 = 2.89 μg/ml

The flux without enhancer is

J = P_{HA}[HA] + P_{A^-}[A$^-$]

= (3.62 x 10^{-3} cm^2/hr)(2.89 μg)

+ (2.19 x 10^{-5} cm^{-2}/hr)(913.71 μg)

= 0.0305 μg/(cm^2 hr)

(b) After treatment with the enhancer:

J = (3.90 x 10^{-3} cm^2/hr)(2.89 μg)

+ (7.97 x 10^{-4} cm^{-2}/hr)(913.71 μg)

= 0.739 μg/(cm^2 hr)

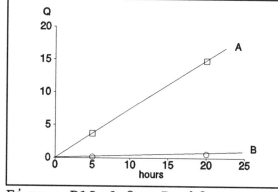

Figure P19–6 for Problem 19.23

(c) Figure P19 – 6 shows a plot of amount penetrated against time (hours) of indomethacin with enhancer (A) and indomethacin without enhancer (B). Note the larger slope, i. e. the greater amount penetrated per hour, due to the enhancer.

PROBLEM 19.24. Using equation (19 – 75), $\dfrac{J}{[A^-]} = \dfrac{P_{HA}}{K_a}\,[H^+] + P_{A^-}$

P_{HA} and P_{A^-} are computed from the slope and the intercept of a regression of J/[A$^-$] against [H$^+$]. The data needed are listed in Table P19 – 6.

The equation is:

J/[A$^-$] (cm/hr) = 140.06[H$^+$] + 19.3 x 10^{-5}; r^2 = 0.967

From the intercept, P_{A^-} = 19.3 x 10^{-5} cm/hr

Table P19 – 6 for Problem 19.24.

$[H^+] \times 10^7$	100	10	1
$J/[A^-] \times 10^5$ (cm/hr)	158	48	7.3

From the slope, P_{HA} = 140.06 K_a = 140.06 x 0.0117 = 1.639 cm/hr.
The permeability coefficient of the nonionized form is seen to be much higher than that for the ionized form of the drug. Therefore the nonionized form is favored over the ionized species for skin permeation. See the pH – partition principle (Chapter 13).

PROBLEM 19.25. $\tau = t_1/t_2$ = 1.20/3.90 = 0.308

$$\eta = \frac{(dQ/dt)_2}{(dQ/dt)_1} = \frac{4.73}{12.1} = 0.391$$

$$C = \frac{1 - (3 \times 0.308) + (2 \times 0.391 \times 0.308)}{[1 + (2 \times 0.391)](1 - 0.391)} \times \frac{6 \times 3.90}{10 \times 10^{-4}} \times 4.73$$

= 32315.7 μg/ml = 32.3 mg/ml

PROBLEM 19.26. Using equation (19 – 65) and the data of Example 19 – 18. (In Example 19 – 18, K was 0.1; the value of K is now 0.1 x 100 = 10).

$$\overline{D} = \left[\frac{(2)(0.02)(1 - 0.02)[(2)(14.3) + 4]}{(14.3/10^{-7}) + (14.3 + 4)/(10)(10^{-10})} \right] + (0.02)^2 (10)(10^{-10})$$

$$+ \left[\frac{(1 - 0.02)^2 [(2)(14.3) + 4]}{(2)(14.3)/10^{-7}) + [4/(10)(10^{-10})]} \right] = 7.67 \times 10^{-9} \text{ cm}^2/\text{sec}$$

$$J = \frac{(7.67 \times 10^{-9})(1 \times 10^4 \text{ }\mu g/cm^3)}{0.0020 \text{ } cm} = 0.038 \text{ }\mu g/(cm^2 \text{ sec})$$

PROBLEM 19.27. (a)   Using linear regression of c/(x/m), the dependent variable, against c, we obtain
c/(x/m) = 21.179 + 0.0139 c; r^2 = 0.999
From the slope, $1/Y_m$ = 0.0139; Y_m = 71.94 μg/mg

From the intercept, $1/(b \text{ } Y_m)$ = 21.179;   b = $\dfrac{1}{21.179 \times 71.94}$ = 6.56 x 10^{-4} ml/μg

(b) In protein binding studies, the Langmuir approach may be used to obtain the binding of small molecules or larger molecules (peptides) to the surface of a large particle such as albumin. The method should therefore be applicable to the binding of a peptide, vasopressin onto the surface of the skin.

PROBLEM 19.28. (a) Using equation (19 – 88), the regression involving $(W/W_o)^{1/3}$ and t gives

$(W/W_o)^{1/3} = 1 - 0.042\, t;$ $r^2 = 1.000$

$k = -\text{slope} = -(-0.042);$

$k = 0.042\ \text{hr}^{-1}$

Intercept = 1

(b) $\log k = 0.525 \times \log(0.034)$

$- 0.578 = -1.349; k = 0.045\ \text{hr}^{-1}$

The value agrees with that calculated in part **(a)**. Substituting k = 0.045 in the equation obtained in part **(a)** the predicted values for $(W/W_o)^{1/3}$ at several times are listed in Table P19 – 7.

After 5 hours, $(W/W_o)^{1/3} = 0.775.$ If $W_o = 2.5$ mg,

$$\left(\frac{W}{2.5}\right)^{1/3} = 0.775 \quad \text{or} \quad \frac{1}{3}\log W - \frac{1}{3}\log 2.5 = \log 0.775$$

$\log W = 3(-0.111 + 0.133) = 0.066;$ W = 1.16 mg

(c) For betamethasone,

$\log k = 0.525 \log(0.002) - 0.578 = -1.995;$ $k = 0.010\ \text{hr}^{-1}$

For sulfamethoxazole,

$\log k = 0.525 \log(5.7) - 0.578 = -0.181;$ $k = 0.659\ \text{hr}^{-1}$

For p – aminoazobenzene,

$\log k = 0.525 \log(0.049) - 0.578 = -1.266$ $k = 0.054\ \text{hr}^{-1}$

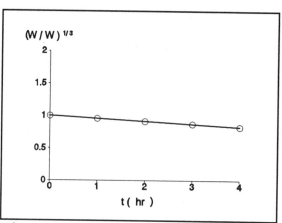

Figure P19-7 for Problem 19.28

Table P19 – 7 for Problem 19.28.

t (hr)	0	1.0	2.0	3.0	4.0	5.0
$(W/W_o)^{1/3}$	1.0	0.955	0.910	0.865	0.820	0.775